J. Centner / A. L. de Weck
Atlas of Immuno-Allergology

ABBREVIATIONS

AA:	Arachidonic Acid
Ab:	Antibody
Ag:	Antigen
AIDS:	Acquired Immune Deficiency Syndrome
ANA:	Antinuclear antibody
BALT:	Bronchus Associated Lymphoid Tissue
BHR:	Bronchial Hyperreactivity
BL:	B Lymphocytes
C':	Complement
CEA:	Carcinoembryonic antigen
CLA:	Chemiluminescent Assay
DNA:	Deoxyribonucleic Acid
DSCG:	Disodium Cromoglycate
ECF:	Eosinophil Chemotactic Factor
ECP:	Eosinophil Cationic Protein
EDN:	Eosinophil Derived Neurotoxin
ELISA:	Enzyme-Linked Immunosorbent Assay
EPO:	Eosinophil Peroxidase
FACS:	Fluorescence-activated-cell sorter (flow cytometry)
GALT:	Gut Associated Lymphoid Tissue
GN:	Glomerulonephritis
GVH:	Graft Versus Host Reaction
GVL:	Graft Versus Leukemia Reaction
HIV:	Human Immunodeficiency Virus
HLA:	Human Lymphocyte Antigen
HRF:	Histamine Releasing Factor
IC:	Immune complex
Ig:	Immunoglobulin
IgE:	Immunoglobulin E
IgG-STS:	Short-term sensitizing antibodies
IL:	Interleukin
IFN:	Interferon
K:	Killer
LAK:	Lymphokine Activated Killer Cells
LF:	Lymphoid Follicles
LT:	Leukotriene
LTT:	Lymphoblastic Transformation Test
Mø:	Macrophage
Mab:	Monoclonal antibody
MAF:	Macrophage Activating Factor
MALT:	Mucous Associated Lymphoid Tissue
MBP:	Major Basic Protein
MHC:	Major Histocompatibility Complex
MIF:	Migration Inhibitory Factor
NABH:	Non-Allergic Bronchial Hyperreactivity
NCF:	Neutrophil Chemotactic Factor
NK:	Natural Killer
PAF:	Platelet Activated Factor
PG:	Prostaglandin
PHA:	Phytohaemagglutinin
PRU:	Pharmacia RAST Unit
RAST:	Radio-Allergosorbent Test
RNA:	Ribonucleic Acid
SLE:	Systemic Lupus Erythematosus
SRS-A:	Slow-reacting Substance of Anaphylaxis
Tc:	Cytotoxic lymphocyte
Th:	Helper T lymphocyte
TL:	T Lymphocytes
TNF:	Tumor Necrosis Factor
Ts:	Suppressor T lymphocyte
TX:	Thromboxane

Jacques Centner / Alain L. de Weck

Atlas of
Immuno-Allergology

Translated from French by Christine de Weck, Dr. phil.

Hogrefe & Huber Publishers
Seattle · Toronto · Bern · Göttingen

Library of Congress Cataloging-in-Publication Data

Centner, Jacques.
  [Atlas d'immuno-allergologie. English]
  Atlas of Immuno-Allergology / translation of French original by Christine de Weck ;
Jacques Centner, Alain L. de Weck. – 3rd ed.
    p. cm.
    Includes index.
    ISBN 0-88937-142-3
  1. Allergy–Pathophysiology. 2. Immunity–Pathophysiology. 3. Allergy–Atlases.
  4. Immunity–Atlases. I. Weck, Alain L. de. II. Title.
    [DNLM: 1. Immunity–atlases. 2. Hypersensitivity–immunology–atlases.
  QW 517 C397a 1995]
  QR188.C4613   1995   616.97–dc20   95-9994 CIP

Canadian Cataloguing in Publication Data

Centner, Jacques
  Atlas of immuno-allergology
  3rd ed.
Translation of: Atlas d'immuno-allergologie.
Includes index.
ISBN 0-88937-142-3

1. Immunology. 2. Allergy. I. Weck, Alain L. de. II. Title.

QR181.C4413   1995   616.07'9   C95-930845-8

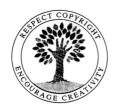

ISBN 0-88937-142-3
Hogrefe & Huber Publishers, Seattle • Toronto • Bern • Göttingen

USA: P.O. Box 2487, Kirkland, WA 98083-2487,
                Phone (206) 820-1500, Fax (206) 823-8324
CANADA: 12 Bruce Park Avenue, Toronto, Ontario M4P 2S3
                Phone (416) 482-6339
SWITZERLAND: Länggass-Strasse 76, CH-3000 Bern 9
                Phone (031) 300-4500, Fax (031) 300-4590
GERMANY: Rohnsweg 25, D-37085 Göttingen
                Phone (0551) 496090, Fax (0551) 4960988

Printed in Germany

TABLE OF CONTENTS

Foreword of the Third Edition

In recent years the tremendous progress achieved in the field of immunology has led to many important practical applications. Consequently a working knowledge of this complex area has become more and more required for a wide range of contemporary health care professionals. Since this field is quite complex, getting acquainted with it can at first be a bit daunting. This is why the present *Atlas of Immuno-Allergology* was created, to provide a reasonably clear and engaging access to this fascinating and increasingly revolutionary field. The success of the first two editions of this book (1979 and 1990) have encouraged the production of a third enhanced version, which, of course, includes the latest information available, and presents a brief discussion of several important concepts from molecular biology, the "twin sister" of immunology.

We thank all concerned for their precious advice, mainly Drs. P. Wynants (Mont-Godinne), M. Bricteux (Eurogentech), J. P. van der Geeten (DPC) Prof. C. Dahinden (Berne) and Prof. B. Stadler (Berne).

This third edition is being published simultaneously in four languages, English, German, French and Spanish. Everyone involved with this entire project would appreciate receiving comments you may have regarding any aspect of the English version, its design, the scope and level of the editorial material, the nature of the graphics, and so forth. We are interested in furthering the understanding of applied immunology, and your comments would help us achieve this goal. Please direct your remarks to the publisher.

Introduction

Immunology is the study of processes by which an organism defends itself against invasion by any foreign substance, however minimal. A major element in this defense mechanism is the ability to recognize "self" and "non-self."

The term "immunity" comprises all reactions whose purpose is to neutralize and eliminate foreign substances. In short, it could be said that an immune response occurs when an antigen encounters an antibody. We shall see that the immune response actually involves several chain reactions. Usually these reactions are beneficial, but unfortunately this is not always the case. Defense reactions can become severely deregulated, and their effect can exceed the initial purpose, thereby leading to inadequate functional reactions and even to organic lesions. These harmful reactions are called hypersensitivity or allergy. In addition, certain elements of an organism itself can become modified (e.g., following a viral attack), with the result that they are no longer recognized as "self." In such cases the organism can react against its own tissues, a condition now widely known as an autoimmune disease.

Immune responses are specific. Upon first contact with a foreign substance the organism learns to recognize this substance through its immune system, which quickly starts a specific defense reaction, aimed exclusively against whatever is provoking the reaction. This invading substance is called an antigen (Ag). In the future, when the same antigen reappears, it is immediately recognized, and the defense mechanism is triggered, via the so-called phenomenon of memory. After a single first contact, the organism is capable of recognizing future attacks by those substances previously dealt with, even though over time this capability might encompass a very large number of antigens. Such immunity is ensured by a series of specialized cells (cellular immunity) and by soluble substances called antibodies (humoral immunity).

The distinction between humoral immunity and cellular immunity is rather theoretical, since the different mechanisms are frequently associated and dependent on each other.

In addition to the defense reactions, a complex non-specific enzyme system, known as "complement" is also very important here.

These various factors and their mechanisms of action will be surveyed in some detail below. Since immunology is a very complex science, we will not hesitate to utilize a variety of simplifications and many graphical illustrations to help explain the key points involved. As we shall see, the text also contains a certain use of repetitions to remind the reader of especially important elements. As a result, you will hopefully find this atlas to be a manageable and interesting introduction to the entire field of contemporary immunology. At the same time it aims to provide an understanding of allergic diseases and the theoretical as well as practical bases for their diagnosis and treatment.

Essentially two goals were envisaged by the authors of this new edition of the Atlas of Immuno-Allergology:

1. To provide a clear and understandable presentation of the key concepts and essential definitions in the field of immuno-allergology for health care professionals, and those still in training, without entering into too much detail, or trying to give a more or less complete survey of the many immunological factors which scientists have thus far identified.

2. To illustrate the text using realistic images, corresponding to the facts which the observer may actually see in the immunological system, be it with the naked eye or through a microscope. In this aspect the Atlas purposedly differs from most modern immunological textbooks, which are heavily based on the presentation of very abstract diagrams.

ACUTE INFLAMMATION

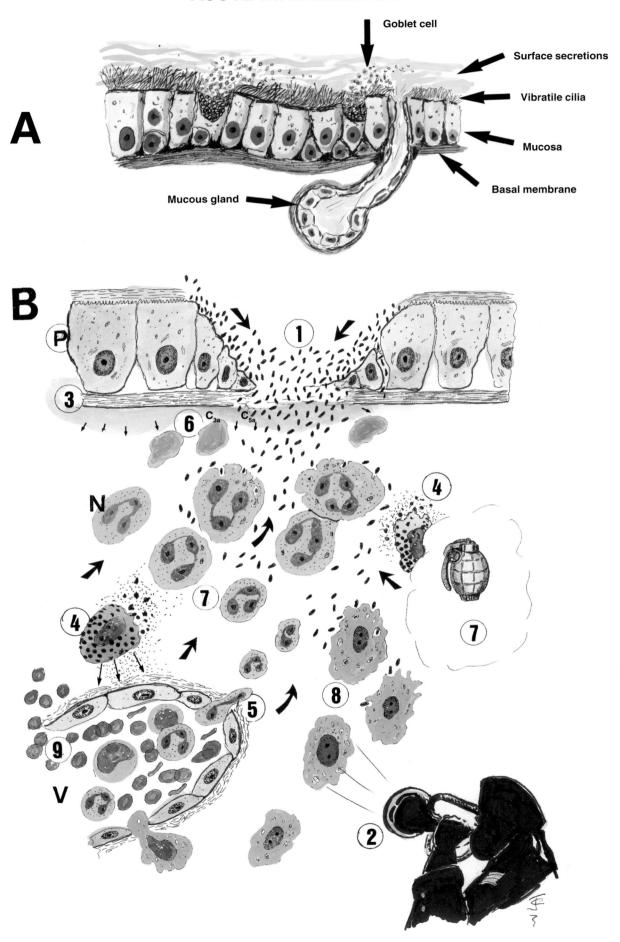

Goblet cell

Surface secretions

Vibratile cilia

Mucosa

Basal membrane

Mucous gland

A

B

P

3

6   C₃ₐ   C₅ₐ

N

4

7

4

7

5

8

9

V

2

Figure 1

Part One

Fundamental Mechanisms in Immunology

1.1 Non-Specific Defense Mechanisms: Natural Immunity

A. Foreign substances are normally prevented from entering an organism by either passive or physical obstacles, such as the skin, mucous membranes, or the mucociliary system. Various secretions from these surfaces, such as gastric acidity, lysozymes, tears, bactericidal fatty acids, sebaceous secretions, and so on, as suggested in **Figure 1A**, play a very important protective role.

B. Once this passive line of defense has been breached, a non-specific reaction, known as **acute inflammation**, very quickly appears, as illustrated in **Figure 1B**.

Acute inflammation is the organism's first line of active defense. As soon as a foreign element, for example a bacterium **(Figure 1B ❶)**, enters the organism the alarm system is set off ❷ by a cascade of mechanisms. The foreign substances (bacteria) activate the alternate pathway of complement ❸, and this activation releases various fragments, which are chemotactic for both neutrophils and macrophages, for example the complement fragments known as C3a and C5a. The mast cells ❹ situated along the vessels degranulate non-specifically at even the slightest microlesion, and upon contact with toxins, microbes, proteases, or other chemical substances. Histamine and other mediators are released, where they first dilate the capillaries and then increase vascular permeability. Liquid filters out of these capillaries as a result, and this "leaking" phenomenon manifests itself as local edema.

In this process neutrophils (N) are attracted towards the site of the invading antigen, which become their target. They have two functions: phagocytosis, and the release of powerful enzymes. Neutrophils are carried by blood vessels (V = vessel – shown in cross section) until the site of invasion.

The first stage of this migration is adherence to the endothelium ❺. Neutrophils then cross the capillary wall due to amoeboid movements, passing between two adjacent cells ❻ and ❼, which appear to retract as the neutrophils pass through. The neutrophils cross the basal membrane, with the aid of a collagenase-type enzyme. They then move in on their target to phagocytose and destroy it. Neutrophils "killed by the fight" become globules of pus ❻. Macrophages catch those invading elements which are able to cross this second defense line ❽. The large-scale migration of neutrophils causes extravasation of a few red blood cells, which in turn cause the microhemorrhages always observed in acute inflammation ❾. In this entire process platelets also play a role in the acute inflammatory reaction.

At the end of this acute inflammatory reaction, if the invader was not eliminated, **the specific immune mechanism** is set in motion with the arrival of lymphocytes, and this produces chronic inflammation.

ANTIGEN-ANTIBODY
(Ag-Ab)

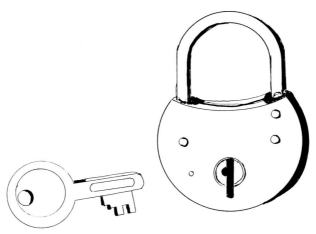

**Image of antigen-antibody complementarity:
the key and the lock**

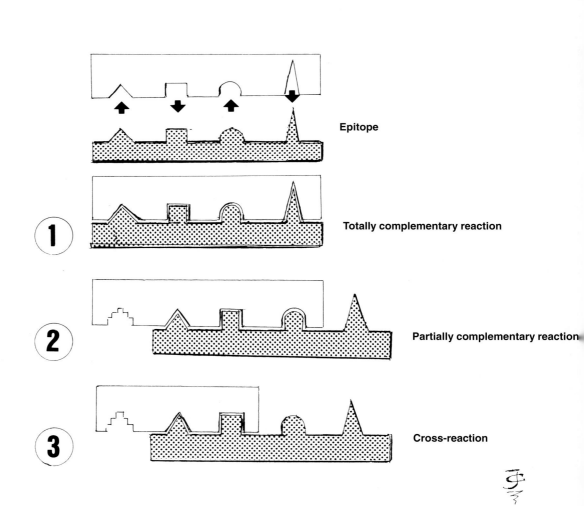

Epitope

1   **Totally complementary reaction**

2   **Partially complementary reaction**

3   **Cross-reaction**

Figure 2

1.2 Antigens and Antibodies

Let us review several essential definitions:
- **Immunogens:** substances capable of eliciting an immune response.
- **Antibody:** a substance (immunoglobulin) capable of reacting specifically with an antigen.
- **Antigen:** a substance capable of provoking a specific immune response.
- **Allergen:** an antigen capable of provoking an allergic reaction, i. e., an exaggerated and abnormal immune reaction.
- **Hapten:** a small molecule, unable to elicit an immune response by itself, but which may do so when linked to a protein. This protein is called a **"carrier protein"** or **"carrier."** Haptens include anorganic substances, lipids, nucleic acids, and certain drugs such as penicillin, etc. The carrier protein may be found in the skin, or on the membrane of a red blood cell, or a blood platelet, etc.

The immune response aims to neutralize, destroy, and eliminate the antigen (Ag). The nature of the immune response is dictated by the stereochemical configuration of the antigen. Antigens are usually large molecules with a molecular weight of between 5,000–100,000 daltons, but sometimes small molecules (less than 1,000 daltons) can also be immunogens, as we shall see later. These smaller antigens are either **"thymus-dependent,"** i. e., proteins with a sequential structure acting on T lymphocytes, or are **"thymus-independent,"** which are usually polysaccharides with spatial structures acting directly on B lymphocytes.

Particulate elements such as bacteria, viruses, parasites, moulds, and red blood cells are all antigens carrying multiple determinants, also called **antigenic sites** or **epitopes.** An antigenic determinant is part of the molecule capable of stimulating formation of an antibody.

The immune response is characterized on the one hand by the appearance of circulating antibodies **(humoral immunity),** and on the other hand by the direct intervention of specifically sensitized specialized cells **(cellular immunity).**

Humoral immunity and cellular immunity may act separately, but they usually act in collaboration, as we shall see throughout this text. Therefore, this differentiation is actually more theoretical than real.

Antibody sites correspond stereochemically to antigen sites. The well-known comparison with a lock and key remains valid **(Figure 2)**. The same lock my be opened with a key that is not exactly of the same shape as the original one. Thus, an antibody might also combine with an antigen of similar structure. These are known as **cross reactions**.

Figure 2 illustrates such complementary reactions: in ❶, we have a totally complementary reaction; ❷ shows a partially complementary reaction, and ❸ is a cross reaction. For example, in hay fever the patient reacts in the same way to different grass pollens, although their antigenic compositions are not absolutely identical. Monoclonal antibodies and the production of recombinant allergens have enabled scientists to establish an antigenic map of numerous pollens, which may provide the means for more specific hyposensitization treatments.

Another example of a cross reaction is vaccination, whereby specific antibodies are stimulated by using killed or attenuated microbes or viruses, or a neutralized toxin (anatoxin, i. e., a modified toxin). The antibodies thereby induced are capable of neutralizing living microbial allergens or toxins secreted by certain bacteria (e. g., tetanus).

An antibody, i. e., an immunoglobulin, possesses in itself antigenic sites capable of eliciting antibodies. These sites are situated either in the variable region and are known as **idiotypic markers,** or in the constant region and are known as **isotypic markers.**

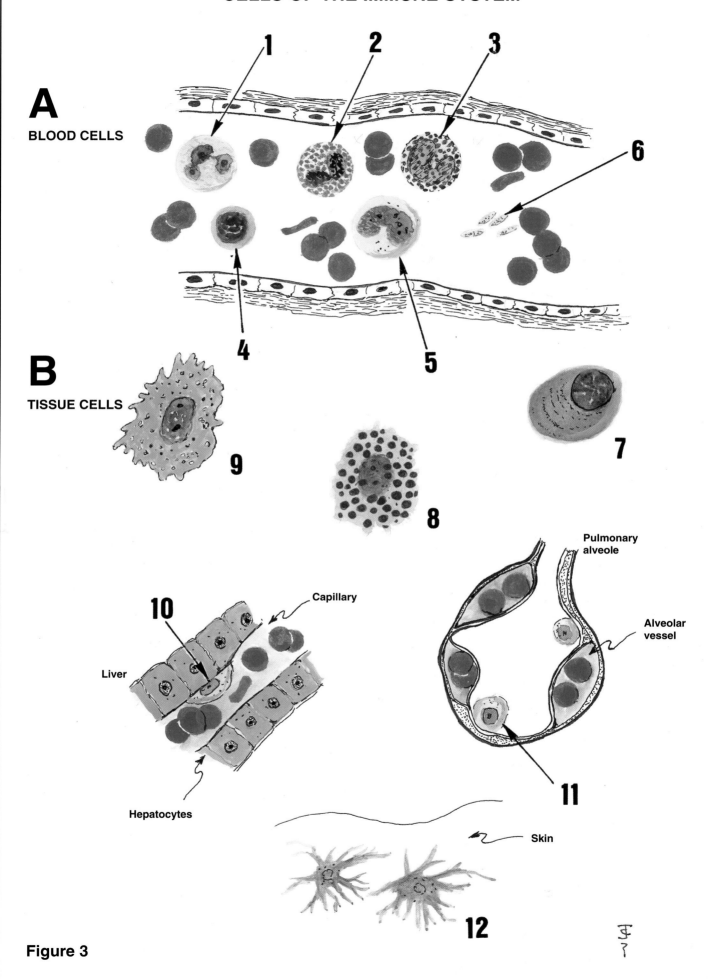

CELLS OF THE IMMUNE SYSTEM

A
BLOOD CELLS

1

2

3

6

4

5

B
TISSUE CELLS

9

8

7

10

Capillary

Liver

Hepatocytes

Pulmonary
alveole

Alveolar
vessel

11

Skin

12

Figure 3

1.3 Cells Involved in Immune Responses

1.3.1 Basic Concepts

As a practicing health care professional, or one in training, you are likely to already be familiar with the basics of hematology, so we would like only to touch on a few main points of this subject relevant to immunology and allergology, and build on this understanding later in further chapters.

Figure 3 shows a kind of family portrait of cells involved in the immune response. **A** shows cells found in the blood: ❶ **Polymorphonuclear neutrophils,** ❷ **Polymorphonuclear eosinophils,** ❸ **Polymorphonuclear basophils,** ❹ **Lymphocytes,** ❺ **Monocytes,** ❻ **Platelets.**

In addition, section **B** shows the cells found in tissues: ❼ **Plasmocytes,** ❽ **Mast cells,** ❾ **Macrophages,** ❿ **Küpffer cells** in the liver, ⓫ **Alveolar macrophages** ("dust cells"), ⓬ **Langerhans cells** in the skin.

The blood cells migrate outside the vessels in order to assume their role. The tissue cells, in contrast, do not normally migrate into vessels; some are even fixed.

The cells of the immune system have two major roles: **phagocytosis** and **mediator synthesis.** Some cells may in fact play both roles simultaneously.

The predominantly phagocytotic cells are the polymorphonuclear neutrophils, monocytes, macrophages, and polymorphonuclear eosinophils. The fixed phagocyte system, known as the **macrophage system or reticulo-endothelial system,** should also be included in this category.

The predominantly secretory cells are the lymphocytes, plasmocytes, mast cells, and basophils; platelets should also be included in this category. These cells, which may release several substances, called **mediators,** turn out to have many functions, but their ultimate task is to destroy invaders. The mediators help other cells to communicate with each other, to transmit orders and to provoke a wide range of reactions. These other cells possess specific **receptors** for these mediators on their surfaces. These **receptors** allow the cells to "hook onto" numerous other cells and biological substances, such as microbes, viruses, hormones, mediators, complement, antibodies, antigens, etc.

Incorporated in their surface membrane, these cells also carry specific molecules having various recognition functions. These are **markers** (frequently designated CD).

1.3.2 Brief description of cells of the immune system

1.3.2.1 Polymorphonuclear neutrophils (Figure 3 ❶)

Polymorphonuclear neutrophils represent 45–75% of the cells circulating in the blood (4,000–10,000 mm^3).

They assume the first line of defense against outside attack, as shown in **Figure 1B**. These cells capture and destroy a number of antigens, especially microbes, by means of enzymes (acid hydrolases, myeloperoxidase, muramidase or lysozyme) contained in their lysosomes (a kind of "mini-stomach") **(Figure 19)**. Lysosomes are seen as dots under an ordinary microscope. When the invader is destroyed, neutrophils often fall victim to their "devotion" and are killed themselves by toxins which they have phagocyted. They are the "kamikaze" cells of the defense system.

These cells are particularly good at intervening in acute bacterial infections, but also in ischemic lesions, in the process of cell elimination, and in necrotic tissue. They can recognize the complex of an antigen bound to its antibody and phagocyte it. Complement fragments C3a and C5a have a chemotactic action on neutrophils which they attract to the site of invasion immediately after intrusion of a foreign substance, as illustrated in **Figure 1B**.

DESTRUCTION OF SCHISTOSOME
LARVAE BY EOSINOPHILS

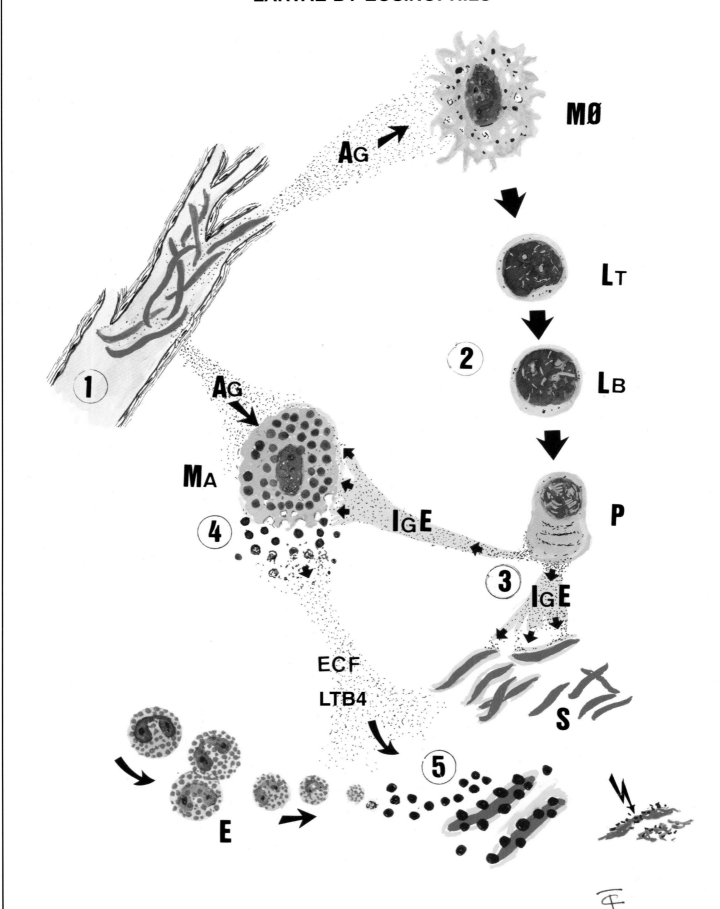

Figure 4

1.3.2.2 Polymorphonuclear eosinophils (Figure 3 ❷)

These represent 2–5% of the leukocytes. Polymorphonuclear eosinophils resemble polymorphonuclear neutrophils, with the difference that they contain large red granulations (eosin staining) and refringent crystals, which may also be traced in the expectorates of asthmatic patients **(Charcot-Leyden crystals)**. Eosinophil counts are increased, especially in allergic reactions, but they also act as a defense against certain parasites, in chronic inflammatory phenomena, and perhaps also in the defense against cancer. Like neutrophils, they do not return to the bone marrow from which they originate, but are eliminated via mucosae.

Since we now have a better understanding of the biphasic nature of certain asthma attacks (an **acute phase** followed, about 6 hours later, by a **late phase**), eosinophils attracted to the inflammatory zone during the late phase are known to cause extensive destruction of the bronchial mucosa. This is fairly similar to the destruction by eosinophils of certain parasites like schistosomes, responsible for schistosomiasis.

As an example, **Figure 4** shows the destruction by immunological mechanisms of schistosomulae (Schistosoma larvae):

Part ❶ shows that after penetration of the skin, Schistosoma mansoni settles in the mesenteric veins, and Schistosoma haematobium goes to the perivesical plexus. From there, they release antigens (Ag) taken up by macrophages (Mø), presenting them to T lymphocytes (TL). These activate B lymphocytes (BL). Area ❷ of the figure shows how these B lymphocytes are converted into plasmocytes (P) secreting specific antischistosomal IgE.

On the one hand, these IgE opsonize ❸ schistosomulae (S), and, on the other hand, they adhere to the membranes of mast cells (M). Schistosoma antigens also come into contact with IgE fixed to the mast cells and provoke their degranulation ❹, releasing various mediators, including ECF (eosinophil chemotactic factor) and leukotriene B4 (LTB4). These factors attract eosinophils (E), which then attach themselves to the schistosomulae ❺ and destroy them.

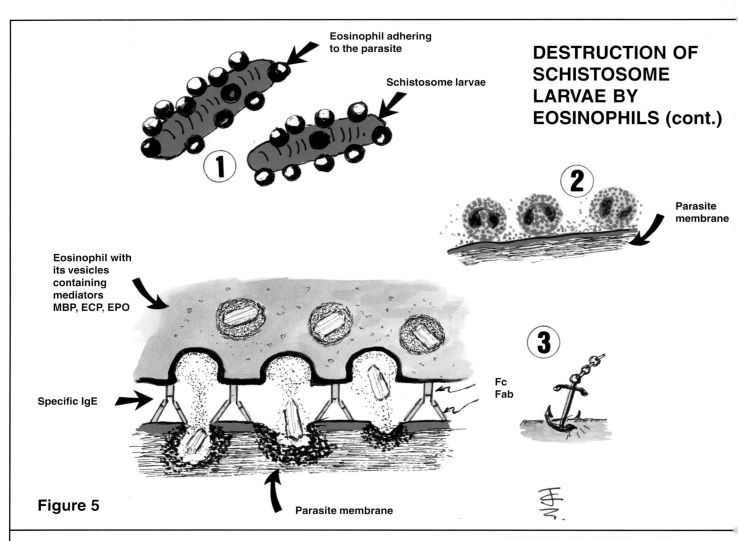

DESTRUCTION OF SCHISTOSOME LARVAE BY EOSINOPHILS (cont.)

Eosinophil adhering to the parasite

Schistosome larvae

①

②

Parasite membrane

Eosinophil with its vesicles containing mediators MBP, ECP, EPO

③

Specific IgE

Fc
Fab

Parasite membrane

Figure 5

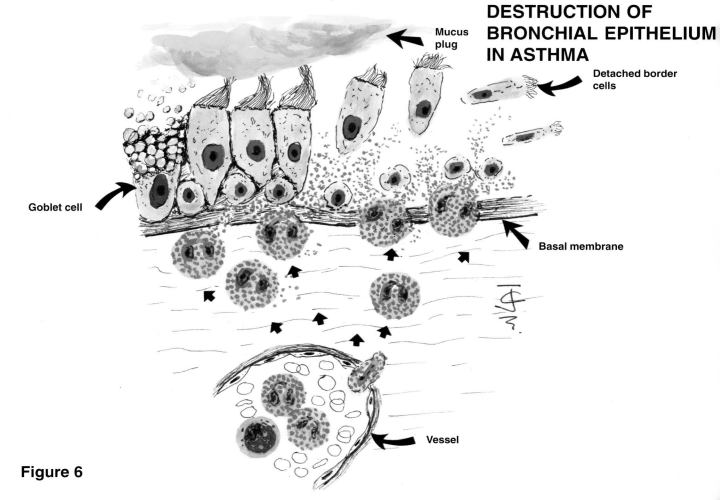

DESTRUCTION OF BRONCHIAL EPITHELIUM IN ASTHMA

Mucus plug

Detached border cells

Goblet cell

Basal membrane

Vessel

Figure 6

Figure 5 illustrates the action of eosinophils. The contact between the eosinophil and the membrane of the parasite is done by specific IgE ❷. The Fab portion attaches to the parasite and the Fc portion fixes to the eosinophil.

Eosinophils are capable of releasing several cytotoxic factors:
- major basic protein (MBP), visible under an electron microscope in form of crystals ❸
- cationic protein (ECP)
- peroxidase (EPO)

From **Figure 5** ❸, we see the highly corrosive crystals penetrate the parasite, and destroy it.

In the late phase of immediate allergic reactions due to IgE, particularly in **asthma**, an invasion of eosinophils **(Figure 6)** attracted by various mediators, including PAF, occurs. Eosinophils migrate from the vessels to the bronchial mucosa, where they release their cytotoxic substances: major basic protein (MBP), cationic protein (ECP), and peroxidase (EPO), as in the destruction of the schistosome larvae. The result is a destruction of the bronchial basal membrane, together with progressive necrosis of ciliary cells beginning with paralysis of the vibratile ciliae. This causes the appearance of mucus plugs for lack of drainage. Finally the necrotic bronchial epithelium is eliminated, leaving the bronchial wall permeable to bacterial and other antigen, as shown in **Figure 6**.

It is at this late and chronic stage that **hypereosinophilia** occurs in the blood.

At present, we recognize and separate several **subpopulations of eosinophils**, according to their density gradient. In this way, **hypodense** and **normodense** eosinophils can be distinguished. These distinct subpopulations seem to correspond to different stages of activation, and are currently under study. Apparently, hypodense eosinophils release MBP from their granules and represent the activated form.

Eosinophils seem to also possess receptors for IgE with both low and high affinity, but in clearly lower numbers than basophils. Probably these receptors explain the eosinophil fixation on parasites covered with IgE **(Figure 5)**. In contrast, the liberation of mediators produced by eosinophils following an interaction between their IgE and a soluble allergen is still not entirely understood.

1.3.2.3 Polymorphonuclear basophils (Figure 3 ❸) and mast cells (Figures 3 ❺ and 43)

Basophils represent only 0.5% of the cells in normal human blood. Their equivalent in tissue are mast cells. Basophils contain large granules loaded with histamine as a main mediator. In addition, when these cells are stimulated, they produce numerous mediators or their precursors: leukotrienes, prostaglandins, SRS, PAF, and others. Normally, these mediators are released when required by the organism. But in some cases they are released suddenly and provoke a type I allergic reaction, such as asthma, urticaria, hay fever, etc. These reactions may even lead to anaphylactic shock.

Basophils and mast cells have on their surfaces a receptor with high affinity for the Fc fragment of IgE **(FcεRI)**. Release of their mediators, the best known of which is **histamine**, occurs either following interaction of IgE fixed to their surface and bridged by specific Ag, or after being triggered by non-specific factors (**HRF** or **Histamine Releasing Factors**), secreted by various cells including mast cells, monocytes, lymphocytes or platelets.

MUCOSAL AND TISSUE MAST CELLS

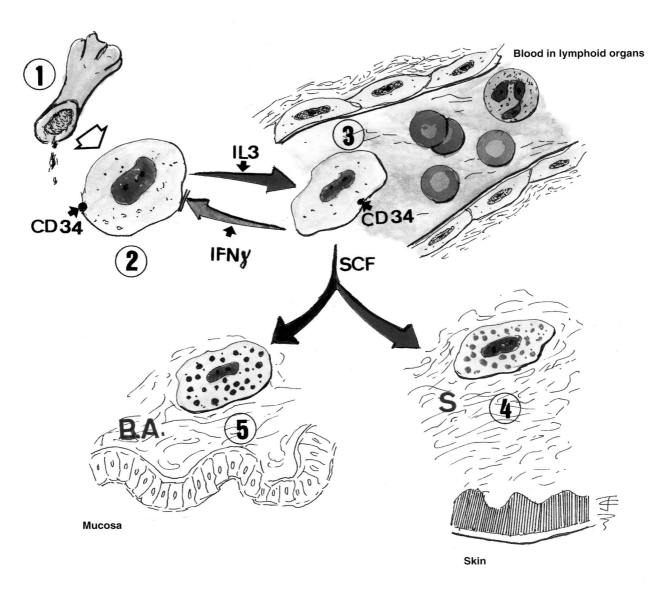

Blood in lymphoid organs

CD34

IL3

IFNγ

CD34

SCF

B.A.

Mucosa

S

Skin

BA: Alcian blue
S: Safranine

Figure 7

Figure 7: There are at least two types of mast cells: **mucosal mast cells (MMC)**, which are abundant in mucosae, and **tissue mast cells** (CTMC: connective tissue mast cell), which are present in the perivascular spaces of tissues. These two types of mast cells are distinguished by the polysaccharide constitution of their granules, which can be seen from their different reactivity with some dyes (Alcian blue, safranine, **Figure 7**). They also differ in their pattern of proteolytic enzymes (tryptase, chymotrypsin). It should be kept in mind that mast cells alone possess tryptase, while basophils do not. Appearance of tryptase in blood after an anaphylactic reaction is a sure sign of the activation and degranulation of mast cells.

1.3.2.4 Monocytes (Figure 3 ❺) and macrophages (Figure 3 ❾; Langerhans cells Figure 3 ❶❷)

Monocytes account for approximately 10% of the cells in normal blood. Macrophages are their equivalent in tissue. Monocytes migrating into tissue are transformed into macrophages. These cells play a major role in the immune system, and have a considerable capacity for phagocytosis. By their receptors they recognize opsonized antigens, i. e., antigens marked and impregnated with specific antibodies. These antibodies play the role of a "sauce" making the antigen more palatable to the macrophage. They contain a large number of lysosomes, which permit them to destroy, modify, or store the antigens.

Through their surface receptors they present the antigen to the lymphocyte, which will trigger either the beneficial or the harmful immune mechanism, shown in **Figure 19**. The recognition of the monocyte by the lymphocyte is conditioned by the presence of membrane antigen on the monocyte belonging to the HLA (human leucocyte antigens) histocompatibility complex.

Certain phagocytotic cells, which can destroy passing antigens, form part of the fixed macrophage system. These include Küpffer cells in the liver **(Figure 3 ❿)**, alveolar macrophages in the lung **(Figure 3 ❶❶)**, and Langerhans cells in the skin **(Figure 3 ❶❷)**, which act as macrophages. These are all dendritic cells. They possess so-called Birbeck granules, deriving probably from invaginations of the plasma membrane.

1.3.2.5 Lymphocytes (Figure 3 ❹)

Lymphocytes make up 10–15% of the normal cell population in blood. They are round and smaller than the other blood cells, with a large, dense, and coarsely structured nucleus and a fine protoplasm. Lymphocytes differ from the cells mentioned above in that they may react directly with an antigen and synthesize specific mediators. Like a computer, they may store information on the antigens they have encountered, via the **memory function** of the lymphocyte, and therefore they play a very major role in the immune system. These cells are mobile but do not phagocyte.

Lymphocytes divide into two groups when leaving the bone marrow: one group migrates towards thymus and leaves it as **T lymphocytes**; the other group migrates directly towards the lymphoid organs: these are the **B lymphocytes**, which acquire certain specific characteristics in the bone marrow. About 80% of circulating lymphocytes have a remarkably long life span: usually measured in months, sometimes even years. The B and T lymphocytes are able to recognize their antigen, due to surface receptors.

Lymphocytes synthesize a large number of mediators, known as **lymphokines**. They collaborate with each other and with other cells, such as macrophages.

T lymphocytes do not produce antibodies, but may produce mediators capable of destroying certain targets (see interleukins). They are divided into several subpopulations:

- **Ts lymphocytes** (also known as suppressor lymphocytes), with depressive or retarding action
- **Th lymphocytes**, which are "helper" or "auxiliary" lymphocytes, and have a stimulating action
- **Cytotoxic lymphocytes** (Tc), which are related to Ts lymphocytes.

B lymphocytes remain under the control of T lymphocytes, which present antigen to them. They are stimulated by Th lymphocytes but inhibited by Ts lymphocytes. T lymphocytes act by means of mediators which include interleukins 4, 5, 6, 10, and 13, among others.

Unfortunately, the various lymphocytes with their very different functions cannot be distinguished under an optical microscope.

MAIN SUBPOPULATIONS
OF T LYMPHOCYTES

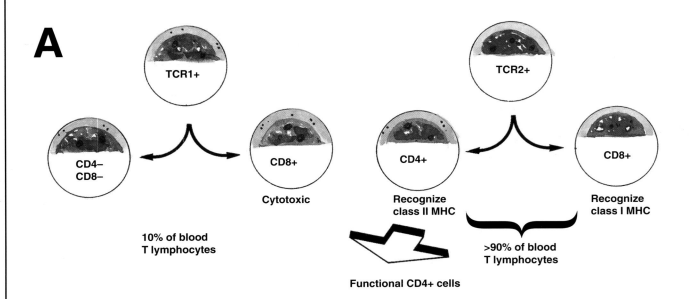

A

TCR1+

CD4–
CD8–

CD8+

Cytotoxic

10% of blood
T lymphocytes

TCR2+

CD4+

Recognize
class II MHC

CD8+

Recognize
class I MHC

>90% of blood
T lymphocytes

Functional CD4+ cells

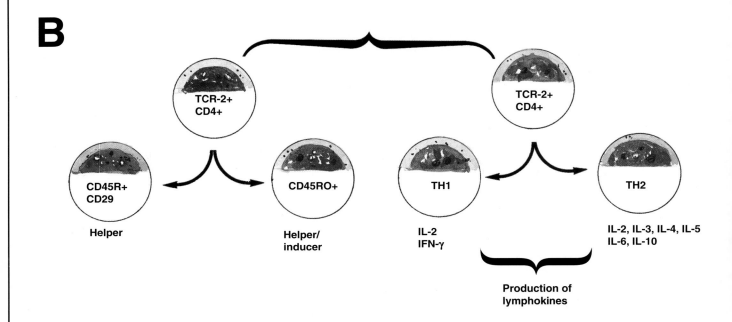

B

TCR-2+
CD4+

TCR-2+
CD4+

CD45R+
CD29

CD45RO+

TH1

TH2

Helper

Helper/
inducer

IL-2
IFN-γ

IL-2, IL-3, IL-4, IL-5
IL-6, IL-10

Production of
lymphokines

Figure 8

Nowadays, the distinction among them is made instead by the use of monoclonal antibodies, which can recognize specific proteins or markers on the lymphocyte's surface. For example, the **Th** react with OKT4 antibodies and the marker is called **CD4**. Antibodies recognizing **Ts** are named OKT8, and the marker is called **CD8**. All T lymphocytes carry CD3 receptors (CD: Cluster of Differentiation) recognized by the OKT 3 antibody.

As shown in **Figure 8 A**, the T lymphocytes subdivide according to their specific receptors (**TCR:** T Cell Receptors), which are composed either of chain α and β (TCR2), or of chain γ and δ (TCR1). The former may generate CD4 lymphocytes, which serve an essentially helper function, or CD8 lymphocytes, which have suppressor or cytotoxic functions. TCR 1 lymphocytes, on the other hand, generate mainly cytotoxic lymphocytes carrying either the CD8 marker or neither CD8 nor CD4. Another basic difference between CD4 and CD8 lymphocytes is the nature of the major histocompatibility antigens (MHC) which they recognize on antigen-presenting cells: CD4 lymphocytes recognize MHC molecules of class II, while CD8 lymphocytes recognize MHC molecules of class I.

Helper CD4 lymphocytes also subdivide into three functional categories, according to the pattern of lymphokines they are able to produce, as suggested in **Figure 8 B**.

While Th0 lymphocytes produce a wide range of cytokines, Th1 lymphocytes essentially produce the cytokines IL-2 and IFN, whereas lymphocytes Th2 produce, aside from IL-2, the "pro-allergic" cytokines IL-4, IL-3, IL-5, IL-6 and IL-10 as well.

The distinction between these subclasses of CD4 helper lymphocytes has so far been strictly functional and seems not to be linked to fixed membrane markers, which would permit their identification by flow cytometry. The range of cytokines produced by T lymphocytes seems to be decisive for the determination of the kind of inflammation provoked by the immunological defense reaction against bacteria, viruses, or any antigen **(Figure 49)**.

Two other types of cells should be added to B and T lymphocytes: the **K or "killer" lymphocytes**, and the **NK** or **"natural killer" lymphocytes**. Remarkably, the origin of these latter cells, which are cytotoxic, is still not clearly understood. The K cells participate specifically, and the NK cells non-specifically, in the destruction of any foreign cell, including bacteria, viruses, or abnormal cells such as cancer cells. It is now well known that **Interferon** γ stimulates the activity of the NK cells. Neutral lymphocytes (T0), neither T or B, also exist.

Lymphocytes form large groups in the peripheral lymphoid organs (ganglions, spleen, Peyer's patches, etc.) where specific areas are reserved for them. The B lymphocytes migrate into zones called "thymus-independent," and T lymphocytes into zones called "thymus-dependent."

Stimulated B lymphocytes are transformed into **plasmocytes (Figure 3 ❼)**, which secrete immunoglobulins. These are cells with a large excentric nucleus. The cytoplasm contains a highly developed and strongly basophilic, granular, endoplasmic reticulum, which is in fact an "immunoglobulin factory".

1.3.2.6 Blood platelets (Figure 3 ❾).

In every mm^3 of blood, there are about 300,000 platelets, which originate from megakaryocytes in the bone marrow. They play an important role not only in the coagulation of blood, but probably also in inflammation, especially in the late phase of asthma. They are stimulated by an important mediator called PAF (platelet activating factor). Platelets survive for about 2 to 3 days.

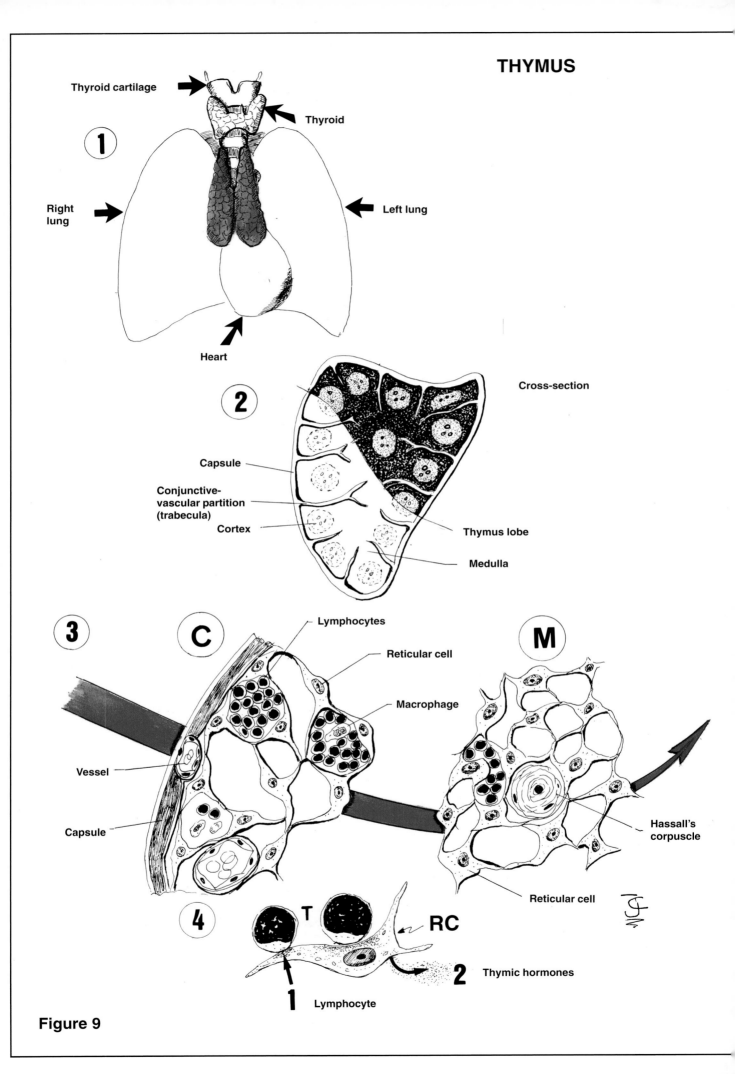

THYMUS

1
- Thyroid cartilage
- Thyroid
- Right lung
- Left lung
- Heart

2 Cross-section
- Capsule
- Conjunctive-vascular partition (trabecula)
- Cortex
- Thymus lobe
- Medulla

3 **C** **M**
- Lymphocytes
- Reticular cell
- Macrophage
- Vessel
- Capsule
- Hassall's corpuscle
- Reticular cell

4
- T
- RC
- 1 Lymphocyte
- 2 Thymic hormones

Figure 9

1.4 Lymphoid Organs

It will be useful at this point to characterize and distinguish the major lymphoid organs, including the **thymus**, which is the central element, and the peripheral lymphoid organs: **lymphatic ganglions, spleen, Peyer's patches, tonsils** and **appendix**.

1.4.1 Thymus

The thymus is a bilobate organ situated in the anterior mediastinum, between the lungs **(Figure 9 ❶)**. In gastronomy it is for better or for worse known as "sweetbread."

The thymus is regarded as an endocrine gland, and secretes various **thymic hormones**. It is composed of lobules **(Figure 9 ❷)** contained in a conjunctive capsule divided by conjunctivo-vascular partitions. Each lobule is situated between two partitions open towards the center. It is composed of a central part, the **medulla**, ❷ and ❸, M, surrounded by a peripheral area or cortex, ❷ and ❸, C. Formations of cells arranged like onion rings are found throughout the medulla, and are known as **Hassall's corpuscles** ❸, which are characteristic of the thymus, but their role is remarkably still unknown.

The thymus is the true "military academy" of the lymphocyte. The prolymphocytes penetrate the parenchyma via vessels completely isolated from the thymus parenchyma ❸, C. The lymphocytes pass directly through the endothelium preventing certain elements of the organism (red blood cells, for example) from interfering with the conditioning of future T-lymphocytes, since this could increase the risk of autoimmune disease. In addition, there are macrophages preventing any foreign elements (such as bacteria) from penetrating into the thymus.

The determining element of the thymus appears to be the **network of reticular cells (RC), the key tissue of immunity, ❸** and **❹**, which forms the body of the organ. Thymocytes or thymus lymphocytes enter into close contact with these cells, containing vesicles of glycoproteins (hormones). Multiplication, differentiation and the start of maturation with **recognition of "self,"** also take place here When the lymphocyte is mature, it only recognizes elements of that body to which it belongs.

While staying in the thymus, a number of **receptors** and **membrane Ag** (markers) appear on the lymphocyte membranes, which enable a differentiation of lymphocytes. Thanks to them, peripheral lymphocytes may recognize the tissues and penetrate them.

It is believed that lymphocytes or thymocytes pass from the cortex (C) into the medulla (M) ❷ and **Figure 9 ❸**, where they undergo further improvements and a final sorting. Ultimately, only a small number of "certified" T lymphocytes will leave the thymus. In contrast to the medullary zone, the cortical zone is very sensitive to X-rays and to corticosteroids, but it manages to reappear quickly if damaged. In humans, the thymus tends to atrophy progressively with time, indeed beginning already at 10 to 12 years of age. By this time, all peripheral organs have been provided with T-lymphocytes capable of dividing and completing their specificity. They migrate continually throughout the whole body, doing their duty as guards against invaders.

LYMPH NODES

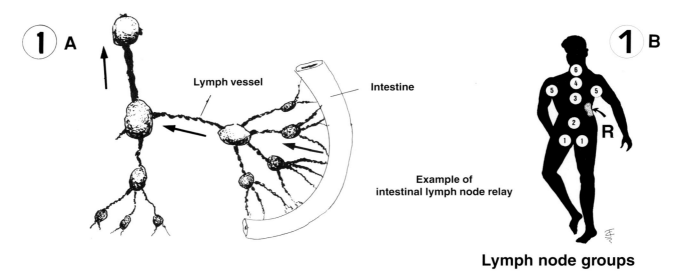

1 A

Lymph vessel

Intestine

Example of
intestinal lymph node relay

1 B

R

Lymph node groups

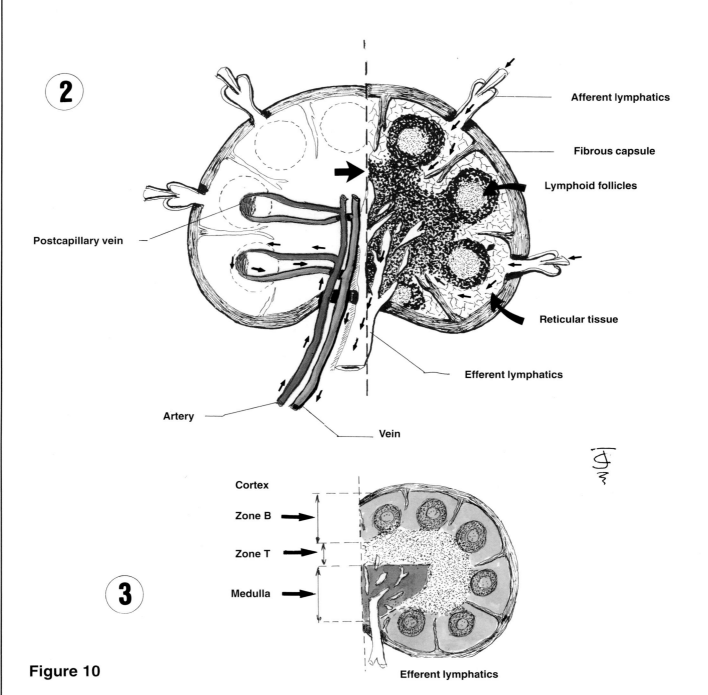

2

Afferent lymphatics

Fibrous capsule

Lymphoid follicles

Postcapillary vein

Reticular tissue

Efferent lymphatics

Artery

Vein

3

Cortex

Zone B

Zone T

Medulla

Efferent lymphatics

Figure 10

1.4.2 Lymph nodes

Lymph nodes are set at all crossroads where lymph is drained, after arriving from peripheral areas **(Figure 10, 1B)**. The principal node groups drain:
- lymphatics of the lower extremities ❶
- lymph nodes of the pelvis ❷
- lymph nodes of the abdomen ❸
- lymph nodes of the thorax ❹
- lymph nodes of the upper limbs ❺
- lymph nodes of the head and the neck ❻.

A lymph node **(Figure 10, ❷)** has the volume of a garden pea, and is surrounded by a fibrous capsule containing lymphoid follicles (LF), separated by extensions of the capsule. These follicles are situated in the outer part of the ganglion and form the **cortex (Figure 8 ❸)**, where the majority of B lymphocytes develop. This is **zone B**, also called the **"thymus-independent"** zone because lymphocytes present there have not passed through the thymus. When antigen stimulation occurs (e. g., the arrival of bacteria via the afferent lymphatics), the center of these follicles, called **germinal center**, becomes hypertrophic.

The **T** or **"thymus-dependent"** zone (containing a majority of T lymphocytes) is located under **zone B (Figure 10, ❸)**.

The guiding of T and B lymphocytes towards their respective areas is referred to as the phenomenon of **"homing."**

The **medulla** lies between the T zone and the hilum **(Figure 10 ❸)**.

Figure 11 ❶ shows details of the cortex of the node. **Reticular tissue** is found between the capsule and the lymphoid formations, which acts as a filter where antigens, lymphocytes, and phagocytes (mainly macrophages) meet, coming from the lymph system. Lymphocytes are probably sensitized to antigens in these perifollicular tissues, and B lymphocytes multiply in these follicles. The mechanisms involved, especially those of T lymphocytes, are unfortunately not yet known in detail. We do know, however, that **antigens are phagocytosed, antibodies are formed,** and **lymphocytes are sensitized mainly in the ganglions**.

The lymph node is the spot where lymph meets blood **(Figure 10 ❷)**. The lymph node is provided with two circulatory systems: one brings lymph from peripheral regions via the afferent lymphatics. Lymph passes through the node, where it becomes enriched in new and sensitized lymphocytes, whereupon it leaves the node at the hilum via efferent lymphatics. The other system consists of an artery **(Figure 10 ❷)**, entering the hilum, branching into each follicle, transforming into capillaries and then into veins, and leaves again via the hilum.

In the region of postcapillary veins **(Figure 11 ❶)**, lymphocytes pass through the venous endothelial wall and migrate toward the parenchyma or directly towards the efferent lymphatic trunk, where they mix with lymphocytes formed in the lymph node. This system ensures that there is a continuous circulation of lymphocytes.

CORTEX OF LYMPH NODE

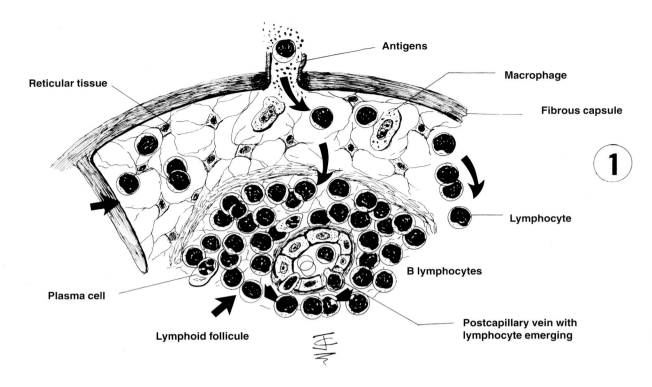

Antigens

Macrophage

Fibrous capsule

Reticular tissue

1

Lymphocyte

B lymphocytes

Plasma cell

Postcapillary vein with
lymphocyte emerging

Lymphoid follicule

SPLEEN

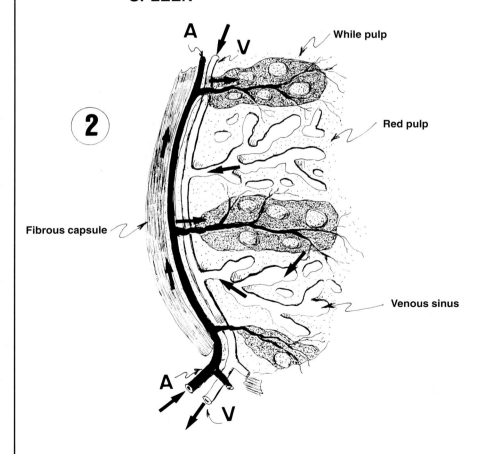

A V

While pulp

2

Red pulp

Fibrous capsule

Venous sinus

A

V

Figure 11

1.4.3 Spleen

The spleen is a large lymphatic ganglion situated in a bypass of the general circulatory system **(Figure 11, ❷)**. Remarkably, it has no lymph circulation. Blood enters the spleen through the splenic artery (A), which branches in the fibrous capsule surrounding the organ. The arterial branches penetrate the periarterial lymphoid formations and follicles constituting the white pulp. This is equivalent to zone B of the ganglions. The vessels end in the reticular zone (red pulp), containing a number of venous sinuses and phagocytic cells.

Immunocompetent antibodies and lymphocytes are synthesized in the spleen, as they are in the lymph node.

In addition to its immunological role, the spleen also has the task of destroying aged erythrocytes.

PEYER'S PATCHES, M CELL

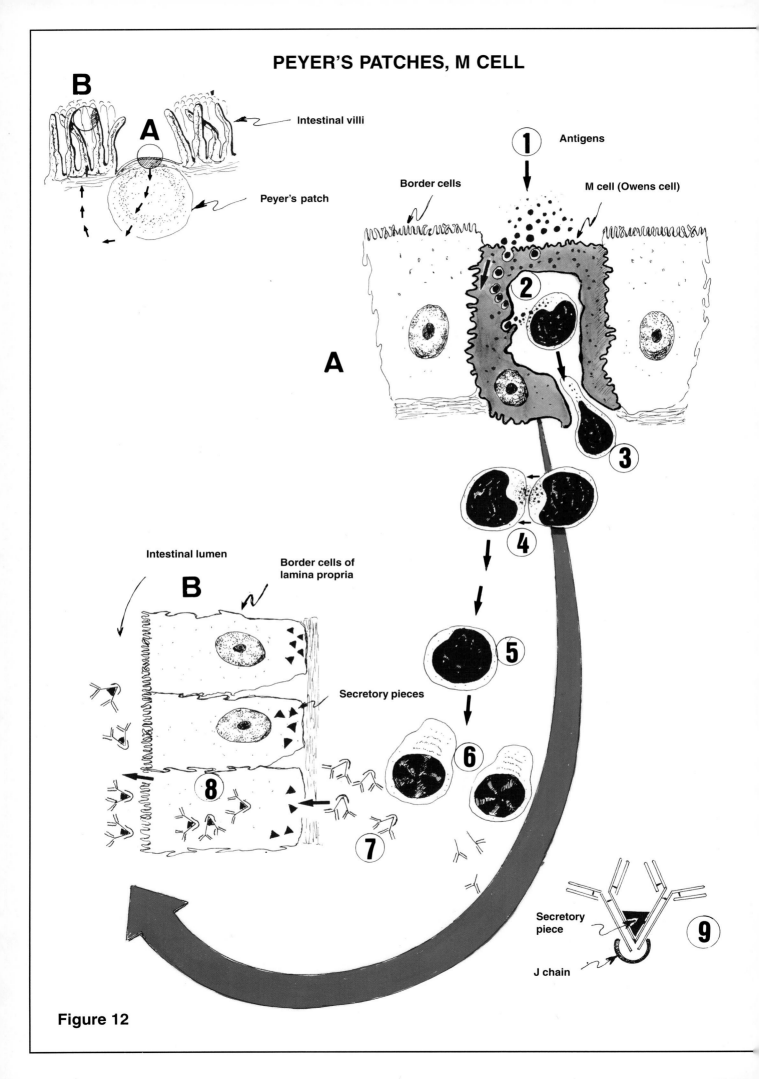

B

Intestinal villi

A

Peyer's patch

A

Border cells

① Antigens

M cell (Owens cell)

②

③

④

⑤

⑥

⑦

Intestinal lumen

B

Border cells of
lamina propria

Secretory pieces

⑧

Secretory
piece

⑨

J chain

Figure 12

1.4.4 Peyer's patches – M cells and other lymphoid organs

Peyer's patches **(Figure 12)** as a whole are a very important lymphoid organ, guaranteeing the defense of the small intestine. They can be as long as 10 cm, and are disseminated in the small-intestinal wall. The patches contain B and T lymphocytes, possess a germinative center and a thymus-dependent zone. Their *modus operandi* is quite interesting.

Peyer's patches **(Figure 13)** ❶ are located within the intestinal villi (small digitaliform formations covering the intestinal walls), as illustrated in **Figure 12** ❸).

Figure 12 shows an **M cell (Owen cell),** among the cells bordering the intestine. This M cell is roughly U-shaped, the bottom of which is directed towards the intestinal lumen, and the two arms point towards the interior of the mucosa.

In ❶, an antigen arrives in the intestine. In ❷, it is captured by an M cell, phagocytosed, and then ejected towards the T lymphocyte which penetrates the arms of the "U." These lymphocytes are continually replaced. In ❸, the T lymphocyte migrates towards the center of the Peyer's patch. In ❹, the T lymphocyte "informs" the B lymphocyte, which will travel a long distance ❺ to finally arrive (as shown in **Figure 12**) in all the intestinal villi, i. e., at some distance from the M cell. Once the B lymphocyte has reached the villi, in the region called "lamina propria," it becomes a plasmocyte secreting IgA ❻.

These IgAs are dimers ❼. The monomer components are held together by the J chain ❾. They penetrate the cell layer bordering the intestine B, combining with the **"secretory piece"** ❾, and pass through the mucous membrane (in ❽) to arrive finally in the secretions of the intestinal lumen. These cells **defend the mucous membranes** (see immunoglobulins A).

CIRCUIT OF B LYMPHOCYTES, PRODUCERS OF IgA

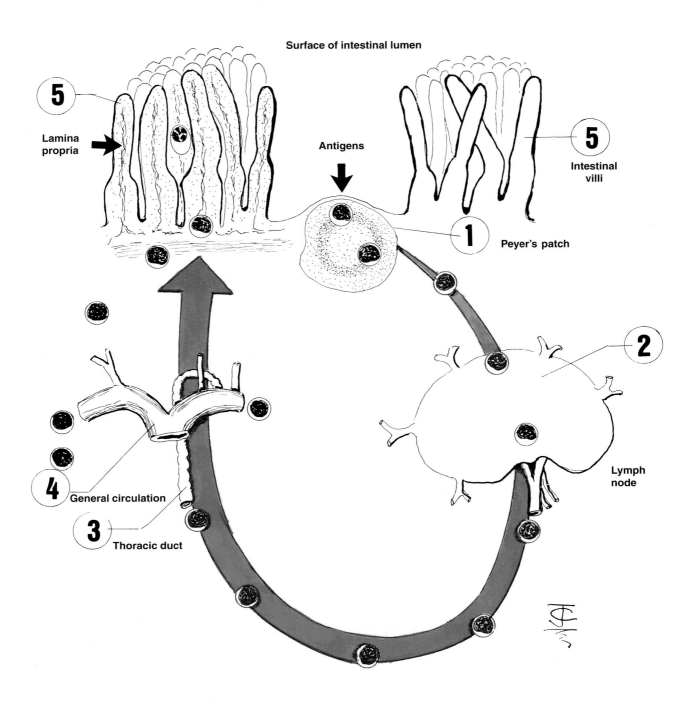

Surface of intestinal lumen

5

Lamina propria

Antigens

5

Intestinal villi

1

Peyer's patch

2

Lymph node

4 General circulation

3 Thoracic duct

Figure 13

The whole of this mechanism is shown in **Figure 13**.

In ❶, the antigen arrives and is captured by an M cell at the level of Peyer's patches. The lymphocytes migrate towards a nearby ganglion corresponding to the zone of Peyer's patches ❷. They pass through the ganglion after having undergone various transformations. Then, they penetrate the thoracic duct ❸, to be discharged into the general circulation ❹. Some of the B lymphocytes travel from here to the different organs (genital organs, bronchi, etc.) and some others travel to the intestinal villi ❺. Once there, they are transformed into plasmocytes secreting IgA antibodies.

In addition to the ganglions, the spleen, and Peyer's patches, the secondary lymphoid organs also include the **tonsils**, the **appendix**, and the many **islets of lymphocytes** situated throughout the organism.

The immune defense mechanism associated with the mucosa is codified **MALT** (Mucous Associated Lymphoid Tissue); **BALT** for the bronchus (B = Bronchus), **GALT** for the intestine (G = Gut), **SALT** for the skin (S = Skin).

CIRCULATION OF LYMPHOCYTES

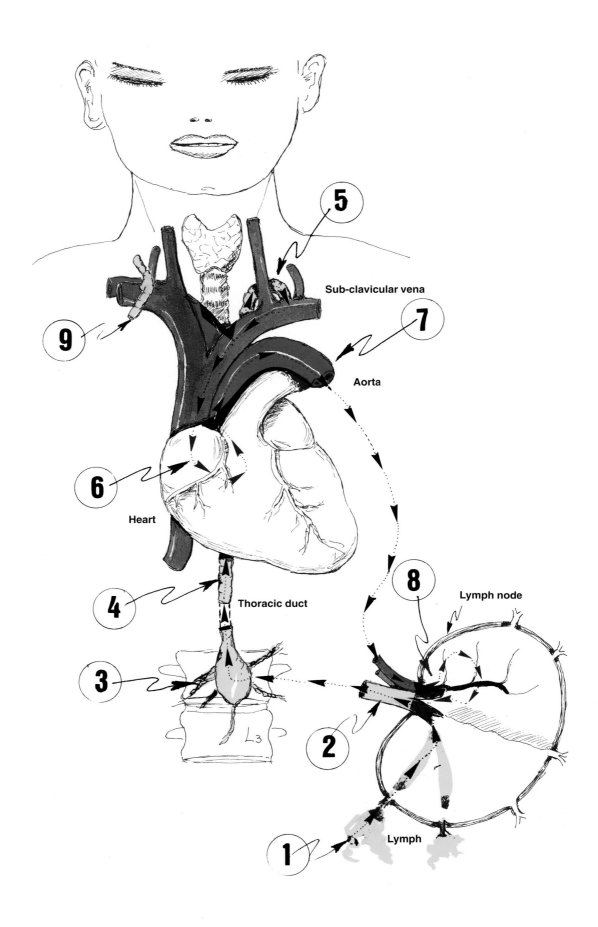

Sub-clavicular vena

Aorta

Heart

Thoracic duct

Lymph node

Lymph

L3

Figure 14

1.5 Peripheral Circulation of Lymphocytes from Lymphoid Organs

Figure 14 shows the lymph coming from peripheral regions carrying lymphocytes and antigens from various local sites, where an immune reaction takes place.

The lymphocytes enter the ganglion via the afferent lymphatics ❶. The lymph, now strongly loaded with sensitized lymphocytes and concentrated in the ganglion, leaves via the efferent lymphatics ❷. The lymphatics meet in what is charmingly known as **Pecquet's cistern**, which is situated along the vertebral column in the lumbar region ❸. From here, the lymph travels upwards in the **thoracic duct** ❹, from where it is discharged into the blood at the level of the left subclavian vein ❺. The lymphocytes are then carried through the general circulation to the heart ❻, and through the smaller circulation to the aorta ❼. From here, they are distributed throughout the body, returning ultimately to the lymphatic ganglions or to other lymphoid organs ❽. In ❾, the big lymphatic vein is shown, which is the draining place of the lymphoid vessels non-tributary of the thoracic duct.

This circulation is continuous. Lymphocytes having entered tissues for some immunological reason re-enter the circulation through afferent lymphatics, and the cycle resumes in this way without interruption.

However, circulatory disturbances may occur, leading either to lymphocytosis, as a result of impairment of the lymphatic circulation, or to lymphopenia following accumulation of lymphocytes outside of the blood stream.

B LYMPHOCYTE DIFFERENTIATION

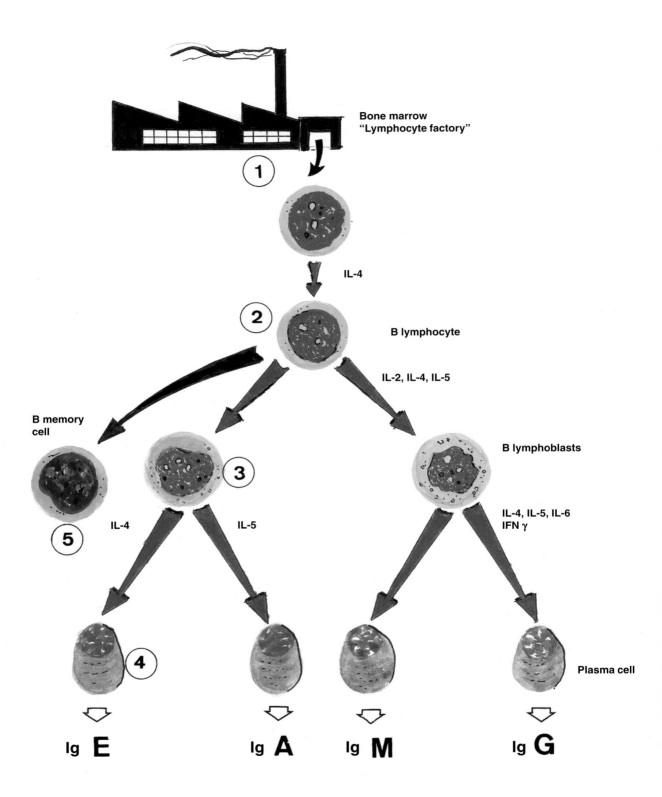

Figure 15

1.6 Transformation and Interaction of Lymphocytes During Active Immune Phenomena

Figure 15 shows the evolution of B lymphocytes and **Figure 16** that of the T lymphocytes.

1.6.1 B lymphocytes

B lymphocytes **(Figure 15)** originate in the bone marrow ❶ (**B:** Bone Marrow) and travel to the lymphoid organs ❷. In humans, they seem to achieve their specificity in the bone marrow, in birds in the bursa of Fabricius. The T lymphocyte cooperates with the B lymphocyte, which after antigen stimulation transforms first into a **B lymphoblast** ❸ and then into either one of two cells: a **plasmocyte** ❺ or a **B memory cell** ❹. The plasmocyte synthesizes immunoglobulins (or antibodies or Ig). Each plasmocyte secretes only one class of specific immunoglobulins, i.e., one antibody against one single antigenic determinant: "one cell – one antibody," according to **Burnet's theory of clonal selection (Figure 18)**. The memory cell stores information on the encountered antigens, which will be used at the next encounter with those antigens.

Expansion and maturation of B lymphocytes into plasmocytes producing a defined type of immunoglobulin IgE, IgA, IgM or IgG essentially occurs under the impulse of an initial triggering signal, which may be the encounter of an antigen in the presence of a CD4 helper T lymphocyte, together with one or the other lymphokines produced by similarly activated T lymphocytes. The presence of IL-4 is important for differentiation into a B cell capable of producing IgE **(Figure 15)**. A more detailed description of the events leading to differentiation of B lymphocytes into IgE-producing cells follows below.

T LYMPHOCYTE DIFFERENTIATION

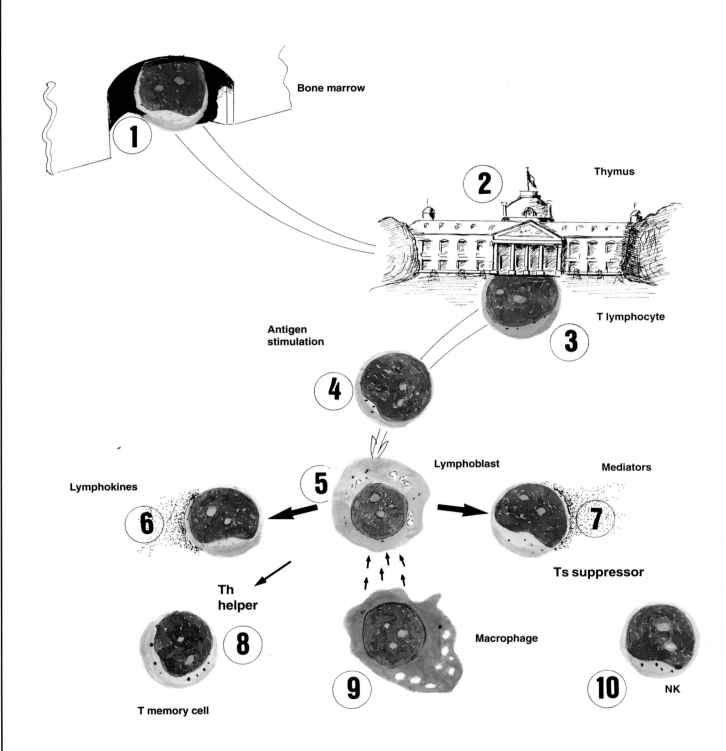

Bone marrow

Thymus

T lymphocyte

Antigen stimulation

Lymphoblast

Mediators

Lymphokines

Ts suppressor

Th helper

Macrophage

T memory cell

NK

Figure 16

1.6.2 T lymphocytes

The T lymphocyte **(Figure 16)** is not yet specialized when it originates from the bone marrow ❶. First, it must pass through the "military academy" of the **thymus** ❷. It then leaves the thymus as a **T lymphocyte** (T = thymus-dependent). The T lymphocyte stimulated ❹ by antigen presented by a macrophage divides into lymphoblasts ❺. Each lymphoblast may give rise to an activated lymphocyte ❻ and ❼ or to a memory cell ❽. During stimulation, the lymphocyte is in close contact with a monocyte or macrophage ❾, which presents antigens and transmits to it all kinds of information required to stimulate proliferation (see interleukins).

Activated T lymphocytes are able to secrete mediators. Some of the activated T lymphocytes are Th lymphocytes (helpers), ❻ and others are Ts lymphocytes (suppressors) ❼. The T lymphocyte is regarded as the "commander-in-chief" of the immune cells. In ❿: **NK** or **"natural killer"** cells are a special category of lymphocytes which are cytotoxic to foreign cells.

Figure 17 shows a synthesis of **Figures 15** and **16**, and summarizes the very effective cooperation which occurs between T and B lymphocytes:

– ❶ Bone marrow, the "cradle" of lymphocytes
– ❷ First step: prolymphocyte
– ❸ B lymphocyte
– ❹ B lymphocyte stimulated by interleukins
– ❺ Differentiation of B lymphocyte into plasmocyte secreting immunoglobulins. This mechanism is "mastered" by T lymphocytes
– ❻ Thymus conditioning T lymphocytes
– ❼ Macrophage capturing antigens and presenting them in digested form to the T lymphocytes;
– ❽ Differentiation of T lymphocytes into ❾ Th (helper) and ❿ Ts (suppressor) lymphocytes. The differentiated lymphocytes secrete multiple mediators (IL and lymphokines) regulating the extraordinary defense mechanism summarily represented in **Figure 17**.

Figure 18 shows the generation of a B lymphocyte clone producing one single specific antibody. The clonal theory is also applicable to T lymphocytes and to their receptors (TCR), specific for antigen **(Figure 21)**.

31

B AND T LYMPHOCYTE COOPERATION

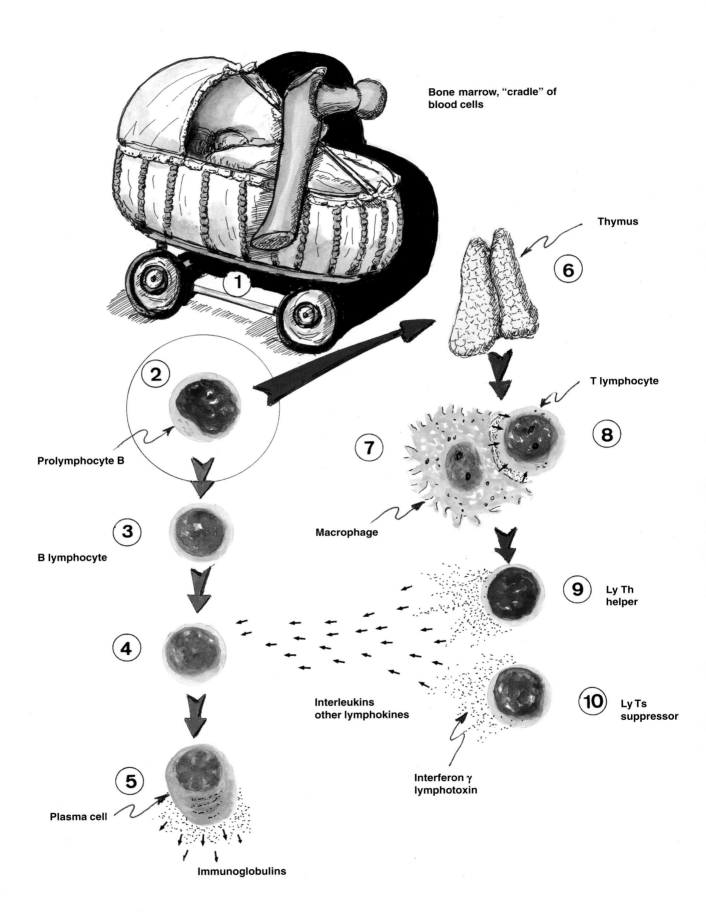

Bone marrow, "cradle" of blood cells

Thymus

T lymphocyte

Prolymphocyte B

Macrophage

B lymphocyte

Ly Th helper

Interleukins other lymphokines

Ly Ts suppressor

Plasma cell

Interferon γ lymphotoxin

Immunoglobulins

Figure 17

BURNET'S CLONAL SELECTION

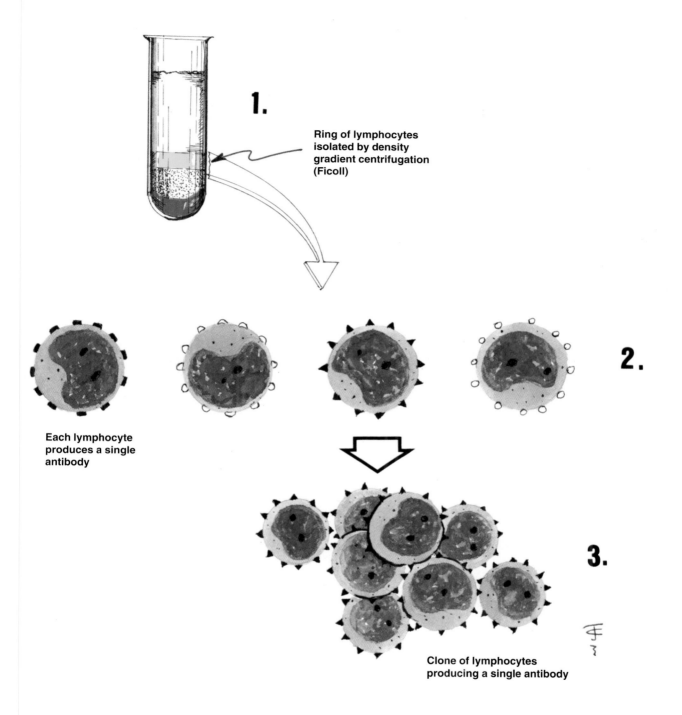

1.

Ring of lymphocytes
isolated by density
gradient centrifugation
(Ficoll)

2.

Each lymphocyte
produces a single
antibody

3.

Clone of lymphocytes
producing a single antibody

Figure 18

MACROPHAGE AND ANTIGENS

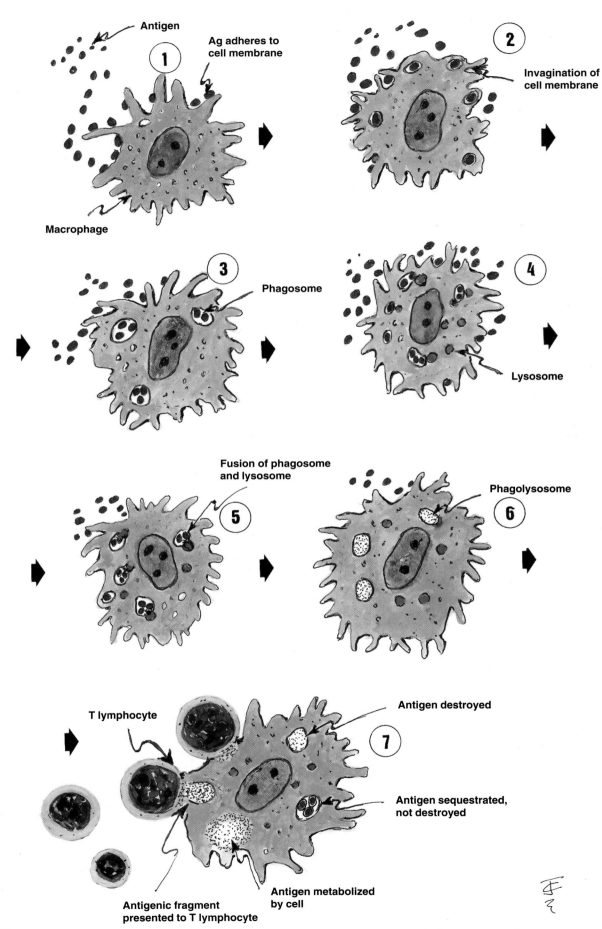

Figure 19

1.7 The Role of Macrophages and Monocytes, their Equivalent in Blood – Antigen Presentation

Macrophages and monocytes are mobile cells, due to their amœboid movements.

Two specific cell types are related to macrophages: M cells in Peyer's patches and Langerhans cells in the skin.

– **M cells**: have already been described with the lymphoid organs **(Figure 12)**.

– **Langerhans cells (Figure 3, ❶❷)**: these are dendritic cells (i. e., cells possessing finger-like protrusions). They contain characteristic granules known as Birbeck granules. They are located in the dermis and epidermis, and are responsible for transmitting the antigenic message to T lymphocytes, probably through direct contact. To help in this function, they secrete mediators capable of attracting lymphocytes. Through their dendritic processes, they form a kind of network enabling them to intercept any antigen which might have penetrated the skin (usually small molecules). They are capable of pinocytosis and, to a lesser extent, of phagocytosis. They have a great affinity for contact allergens and haptens, such as nickel and chromium, and probably play an important role in contact eczema. They also possess receptors for IgE. When stimulated by contact with allergens specific for these IgEs, such as (house dust mites or food allergens), Langerhans cells produce inflammatory mediators and may thus equally cause IgE-dependent eczematous lesions, as encountered in atopic eczema.

Macrophages have a tremendous capacity for phagocytosis and play a major role in the defense of the organism. They are also responsible for the synthesis of a large number of substances, such as lysosomal enzymes, interferon, complement, transferrin, interleukins, etc., and – as we shall see – they collaborate closely with the lymphocytes. They possess many membrane receptors (markers) for Ig Fc, C3, etc.

Macrophages **(Figure 19)** belong to the **"macrophage system"** (formerly the RES or reticuloendothelial system), which includes:

a. **Circulating macrophages**: blood monocytes, macrophages of the pulmonary alveoles, macrophages of the peritoneum and of pleura, etc.

b. **Fixed macrophages** (called **histiocytes, Figure 3**), such as the Küpffer cells in the liver, pulmonary alveolar macrophages, macrophages of spleen sinuses, lymphatic ganglions, bone marrow, microglial cells of the central nervous system, adrenals, pituitary, etc.

The macrophage captures the antigen upon penetrating the organism and digests it in form of fragments which become immunogenic when fixed to the macrophage membrane **(Figure 19)** and presented to T lymphocytes.

Thus, the macrophage presents antigen to the T lymphocyte after digestion and transformation. In addition, it produces mediators which activate the lymphocyte: interleukins and prostaglandins.

Formations called lysosomes are found in macrophages, and can be regarded as "mini-stomachs", as they contain very powerful enzymes capable of digesting a wide range of substances. This digestion serves either to benefit the cell itself, to destroy phagocytosed elements, or to transform the antigen and render it accessible to the lymphocyte. Some lymphokines produced by activated T lymphocytes (e. g., interferon γ) in turn activate macrophages.

Figure 19 shows in ❶ antigens captured by a macrophage, with contact being facilitated by the cell's amœboid movements. Antigen adheres to the macrophage's membrane either following complement activation through fixation of C3 b on the antigen, or through binding of the Fc fragment of an antibody having reacted with the antigen.

OPSONISATION OF Ag

MACROPHAGE AS SEEN IN ELECTRON MICROSCOPE

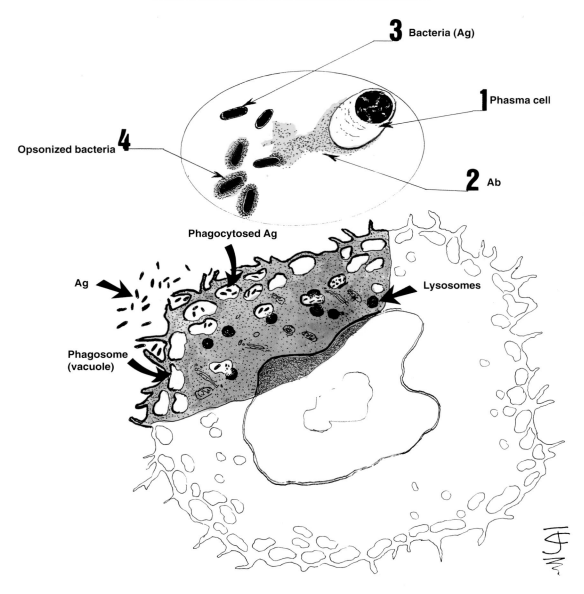

3 Bacteria (Ag)

1 Phasma cell

Opsonized bacteria **4**

2 Ab

Phagocytosed Ag

Ag

Lysosomes

Phagosome (vacuole)

Figure 20

This is known as the opsonization phenomenon, and is illustrated in **Figure 20**. The phagocyte ❷ forms invaginations of its wall around the antigen. In ❸, the antigen is trapped in a vesicle called a phagosome. In ❹, the phagosomes come into contact with lysosomes. In ❺ and ❻, lysosomes and phagosomes merge into phagolysosomes. In ❼, the antigen is digested.

The possible fates of antigen are illustrated in ❽. It might
– be stored in the cell as a metabolic element,
– be presented in the form of a peptide by histocompatibility antigens **(Figure 21)** and put in contact with lymphocytes,

– be stored within the cell when digestion is impossible (as in the case of tubercle bacilli, which are protected by their waxy capsule),
– or simply be destroyed.

Figure 20 illustrates the **opsonization** phenomenon and antigen phagocytosis by a macrophage, as seen under an electron microscope.

Macrophages have therefore **two essential roles**:
1. Attraction and digestion of antigen
2. Presentation of antigenic fragments to T lymphocytes.

MECHANISM OF ANTIGEN PRESENTATION BY MHC

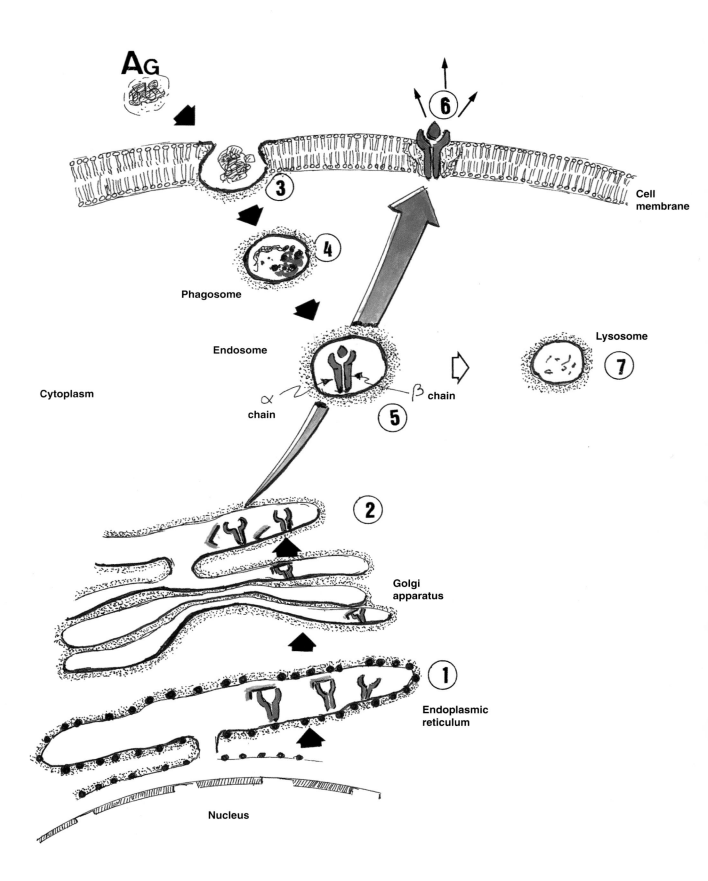

Figure 21A

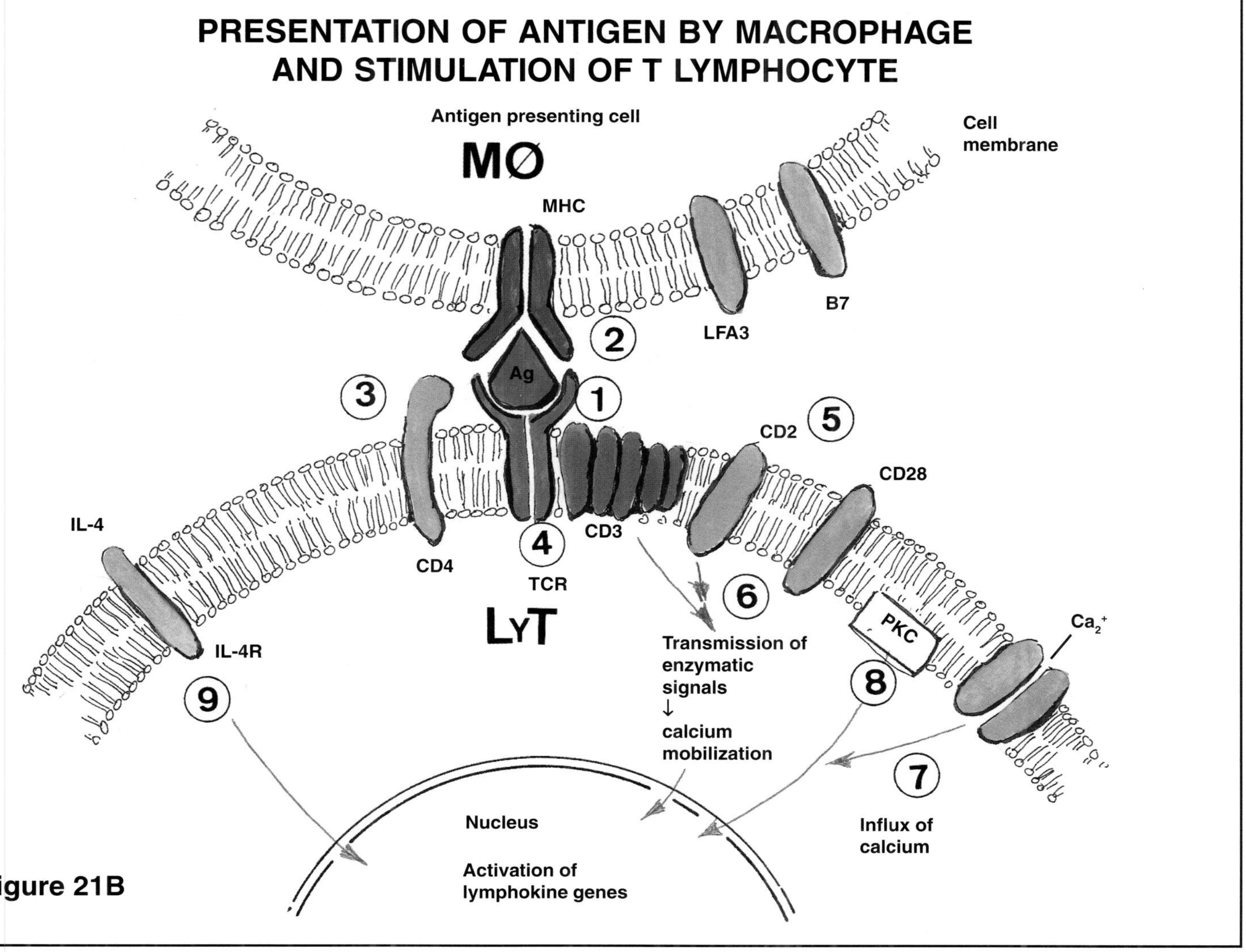

PRESENTATION OF ANTIGEN BY MACROPHAGE AND STIMULATION OF T LYMPHOCYTE

Figure 21B

Figure 21 A. At the molecular level, presentation of the antigen's peptide fragments, after digestion by the macrophage, occurs via the major histocompatibility antigen MHC. This process takes place as follows: In ❶, the two chains α and β of a MHC class II molecule, as well as a protecting chain L, are synthesized in the endoplasmic reticulum. These molecules pass into the Golgi apparatus ❷ in which the protecting L chain is eliminated. Antigen ingested by the macrophage ❸ is then digested into peptides in the phagosomes ❹. Peptides assemble with MHC molecules in an endosome ❺. The complex antigenic peptide-MHC molecule is then expressed on the cell membrane ❻, while other non-used fragments of antigen are finally digested in lysosomes ❼.

Figure 21 B: The specific recognition element, the T cell receptor **(TCR)** consists of two chains α and β. It is as-sociated with a series of molecules collectively called CD3, which are themselves associated with enzymes such as tyrosine-kinase and protein kinase C ❽, which play a decisive role in the intracellular transmission of activation signals, and in the intranuclear activation of cellular genes. A stream of membrane lipids (PIP, IP, DG) ❽ and calcium influx ❼ participate to signal transmission. In T cell activation, interaction with co-stimulatory molecules such as CD4 ❸, MHC ❷ or CD2 ❺ and LFA3, as well as interaction with some cytokines such as IL-2 and IL-4 ❾ and their respective receptors, are also implicated.

In order for macrophages to be attracted by antigen, the latter must be "opsonized," i. e., coated with a specific antibody which will be easily bound to the macrophage's receptors for the antibody's Fc fragment **(Figure 20).**

39

INTERLEUKINES

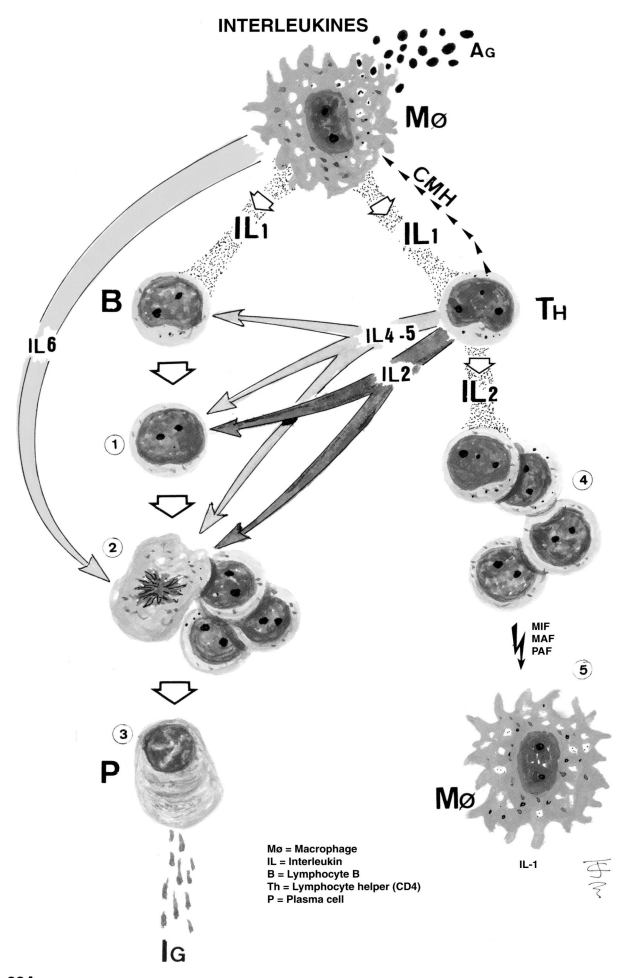

Mø = Macrophage
IL = Interleukin
B = Lymphocyte B
Th = Lymphocyte helper (CD4)
P = Plasma cell

Figure 22A

1.8 Soluble Cellular Mediators or Cytokines

All soluble mediators of cellular origin are gathered under the term cytokines. These are not antibodies, but rather substances released during the activation of inflammatory cells by various stimuli (e. g., other cytokines).

They are called **lymphokines** or **monokines**, according to whether the producing cell belongs to the lymphocyte or monocyte system.

Among lymphokines, some play a major role in the activation and differentiation of **T and B lymphocytes (Figure 19)**: these are **interleukins** (IL). Some of them constitute a growth factor indispensable to assure the survival of lymphocyte cultures, others are indispensable for activating certain functions. When fixed or circulating monocytes or macrophages are stimulated by an antigen or a mitogen (e. g., phytohemagglutinin – PHA), they produce interleukin 1 (IL-1). Lymphocytes which recognize the macrophage, and only those, collaborate with macrophages. They recognize a surface antigen on the macrophages which is a molecule of the **major histocompatibility complex** (MHC).

Figure 22 A summarizes the role of interleukins (IL) in the differentiation and proliferation of lymphocytes. The first step, the meeting of a macrophage with a T lymphocyte, is called stimulation phase. It enables the T lymphocyte to respond to the antigen or to various mediators.

Under the influence of the antigen (or of mitogenic substances), the Th lymphocyte stimulated by IL-1 produces interleukin 2, which in turn causes proliferation of T lymphocytes (proliferation phase ❹). These lymphocytes then also produce lymphokines (such as migration inhibitory factor – MIF, macrophage activating factor – MAF, PAF, etc.) which stimulate the macrophage ❺ in its struggle against bacteria or other antigens. Lymphocytes can also stimulate macrophages to produce IL-1. Let's note here that in contrast, Cortisone and prostaglandins such as PGE2 inhibit production of IL-1.

Some T lymphocytes (Th2) produce **IL-4** and **IL-5**, which stimulate various stages in the differentiation of B lymphocytes. IL-2 can also stimulate B lymphocytes. In addition, macrophages produce **IL-6**, which also stimulates B lymphocytes **(Figure 19)**.

The list of interleukins does not stop here. Since the discovery of **IL-3** (which is produced by T lymphocytes and stimulates bone marrow as well as various other cells), scientists have also recognized many other interleukins, such as **IL-4**, (which is produced by lymphocytes but also by activated mast cells, basophils and stimulated T and B lymphocytes), **IL-8** (produced by monocytes and stimulated neutrophils), **IL-9, IL-10, IL-11, IL-12** and **IL-13**. Others will certainly follow.

Figure 22 A: Mø: macrophage; IL: interleukin; B: B lymphocytes; Th: helper lymphocytes (CD4).
❶ B lymphocyte stimulated; ❷ its division; ❸ P = plasmocyte; ❹ Proliferation of T lymphocyte; ❺ Macrophage stimulation.

Two more cytokines also play a considerable role: **TNF** and **interferon γ**. TNF (Tumor Necrosis Factor) or **"cachectin"** is produced by monocytes and activated macrophages. It is an immunomodulator, which determines cytotoxicity of macrophages, lysis of cancer cells and stimulation of neutrophils.

Gamma interferon is produced by T lymphocytes activated by an antigen or mitogen. Controlled partly by IL-1 and IL-2, it regulates various immunological functions of macrophages, and stimulates activity of some B lymphocytes (production of IgG) but may inhibit the activity of IgE-producing B lymphocytes.

From all this, we can see that cytokines have different and very important effects on **maturation and differentiation of cells of the immune system.**

AGONIST AND RESPONSE MODIFYING CYTOKINES
IN ALLERGIC INFLAMMATION

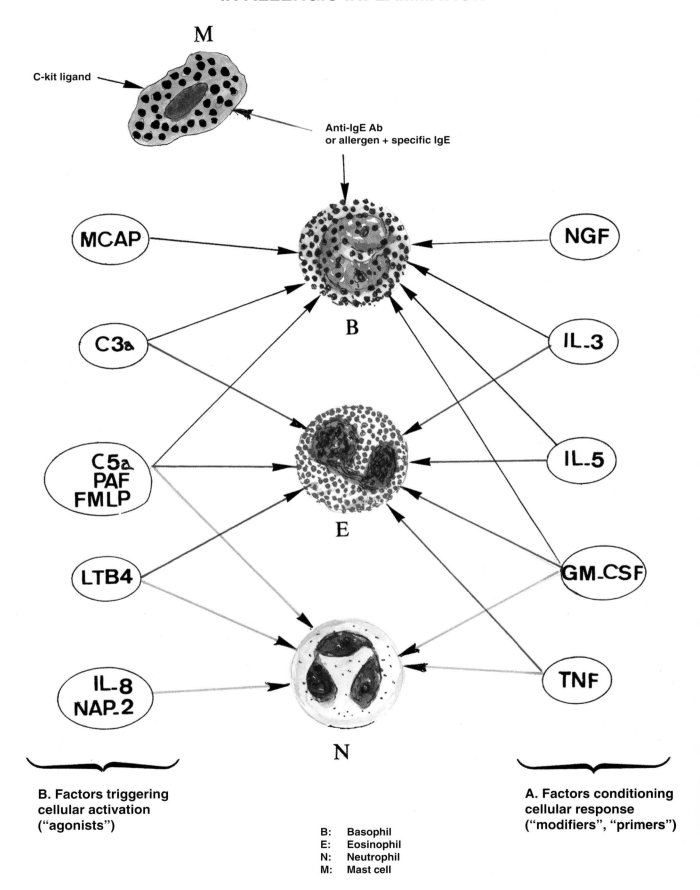

B. Factors triggering
cellular activation
("agonists")

A. Factors conditioning
cellular response
("modifiers", "primers")

B: Basophil
E: Eosinophil
N: Neutrophil
M: Mast cell

Figure 22B

Figure 22 B: Another very important cytokine activity is their **capacity to modify the response of inflammatory cells ("priming")** or to **trigger production/release of inflammatory mediators**.

A first category of cytokines **(Figure 22 B (A))** enhances the response of various blood cells but does not trigger it. These cytokines are factors **modifying the response.** Some lymphokines, such as GM-CSF, act on several cell types, such as neutrophils, eosinophils and basophils, while others, such as IL-3 or IL-5, have a more restricted range of activity. Human mast cells seem to react only to another cytokine, namely "Stem cell factor" or "c-kit ligand." The physical basis of these apparently specific actions stems from specific receptors present on different cell types for various cytokines.

A second category of cytokines **(Figure 22B (B))** is capable of directly triggering the production or release of mediators. Those factors, produced by activated T lymphocytes and macrophages, are sometimes globally called **"histamine releasing factors."** They contribute to the late phase of the anaphylactic reaction **(Figure 48)**, and to chronic allergic inflammation. It should be noted that the capacity to trigger mediator release is not limited to certain cytokines. The triggering agents encompass specific IgE antibodies as well as the complement components C3a and C5a (anaphylatoxins), in addition to the mediators (PAF, LTB4) and various other substances (FMLP, opiates, basic peptides etc.). These non-specific triggers are mostly involved in so-called **pseudo-allergic reactions** which are not triggered by a specific allergen, but which, nevertheless, involve the same mediators and cause the same symptoms as classical IgE-dependent allergic reactions.

IMMUNOGLOBULINS

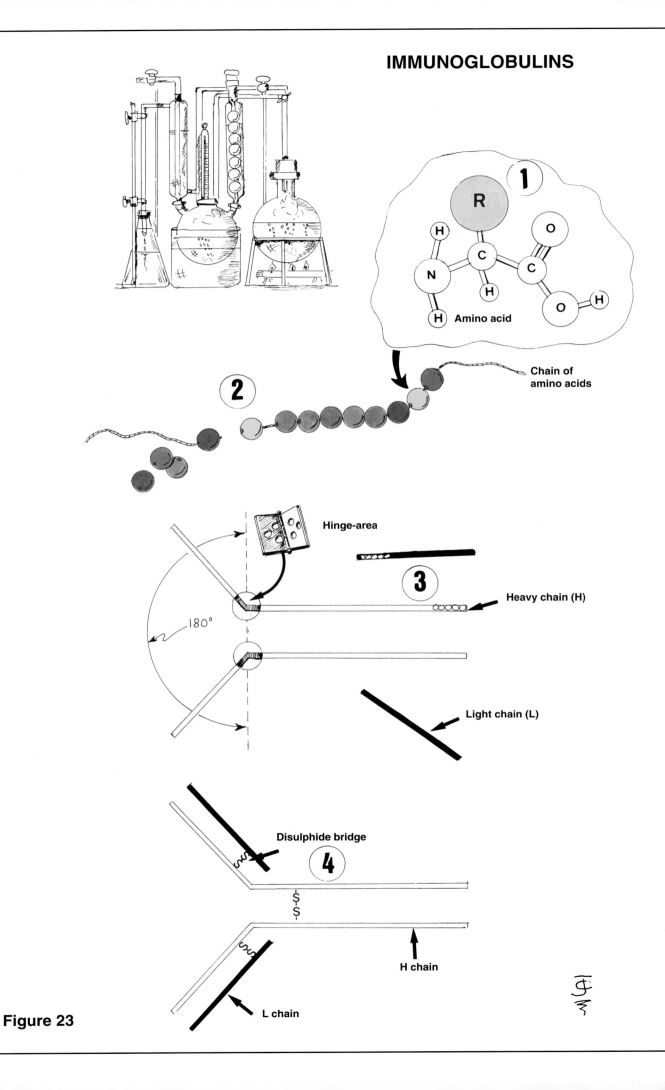

Figure 23

1.9 Immunoglobulins

Unfortunately, the terms **immunoglobulin or Ig** or **antibody (Ab)** are used indiscriminately. All antibodies are immunoglobulins, but not all immunoglobulins are necessarily functional antibodies.

1.9.1 Plasmocytes

B lymphocytes are transformed after antigenic stimulation into **plasmocytes**, which are cells with eccentric nuclei, abundant chromatin arranged like spokes of a wheel, and markedly basophilic cytoplasm.

Plasmocytes synthesize immunoglobulins or antibodies in large quantities and discharge them into the blood plasma.

Antibodies are **specific**, i. e., they correspond to the antigen that has induced their formation. To each antigenic determinant (epitope) of the antigen corresponds a single antibody.

Each plasmocyte synthesizes one single immunoglobulin. Upon immunization, among a large number of plasmocytes each secretes one specific immunoglobulin, so that a mixture of immunoglobulins is found in plasma. Then, these immunoglobulins may be analyzed or extracted.

1.9.2 Structure of Immunoglobulins

Figure 23: Immunoglobulins are composed of four polypeptide chains. **Figure 23 ❶** shows the general formula of an amino acid (R is a hydrocarbon radical). Polypeptides are amino acid chains which may be compared to beads in a necklace ❷. There are two **long** or **heavy** chains (**H** or heavy chain) ❸ and ❹, with each one constituted of some 400 amino acids, and two **short** or **light** chains (**L** or light chain), where each is constituted of about 200 amino acids. The four chains are linked together by disulfide bridges ❹. According to the composition of the heavy chains, the following Igs may be distinguished:

– IgA with an α heavy chain (defense of mucous membranes)
– IgM with a μ heavy chain (early defense against infections, especially viral infections)
– IgG with a γ heavy chain (general defense)
– IgE with a ε heavy chain (reagin allergy), and
– IgD with a δ heavy chain (defense)

Ig may polymerize (2 molecules for IgA, 5 for IgM, etc.) **(Figure 26)**.

Figure 24: The heavy and light chains consist of two parts: a **variable part** (V), shown in red, and a **constant part** (C), shown in blue. The antibody function is situated in the variable part. This portion of the molecule could be described as the "homing head" of Ig as it seeks out the antigen. The variable part could be compared to the forelimbs of a praying mantis **(Figure 25)** or the claws of a lobster.

The primary structure (i. e., the amino acid chain in its simplest chemical expression) of these Ig is conventionally represented as in **Figure 23 ❹**: two H chains and two L chains linked by disulfide bridges. It should also be noted that the H chains possess a hinge zone and may separate from each other by 0–180 degrees, allowing them to adjust to the size of the antigen **(Figure 23 ❸)**.

Since Igs are large protein molecules migrating slowly, they migrate in serum electrophoresis in the gamma zone (see Electrophoresis).

1.9.3 Fab and Fc Fragments

If an Ig molecule is cleft by an enzyme called papain, two large fragments are obtained: **the Fab part and the Fc part (Figure 24 ❷)**. The notion of Fab and Fc fragments is important in practice, as each part has a well defined function. Reflecting this importance, there are innumerable references in the immunology literature to Fab or Fc fragments.

The Fab and Fc functions may be compared to limbs of a praying mantis **(Figure 25)**.

The **Fab part** (forelimbs of the praying mantis ❶ and ❷) is the one to recognize a specific antigen and to fix it. The **antibody site is constituted by an Fab2 fragment**: 2 Fab fragments linked by one or several disulfide bridges **(Figure 24)**.

The **Fc part**, the hind limbs of the mantis, possesses a number of non-specific binding sites, enabling the Ig to fasten itself to some chemical substance, such as a complement component or a cell membrane receptor (Fc receptor), as suggested in **Figure 25**.

The Fc part may also fix a fluorescent dye or a radioactive substance. Thus Ig may be used as a marker (see Immunofluorescence and RAST). Such a marked Ig, while carrying a dye or an isotope, may then, as a second antibody, bind to an antibody or to a protein functioning as an antigen.

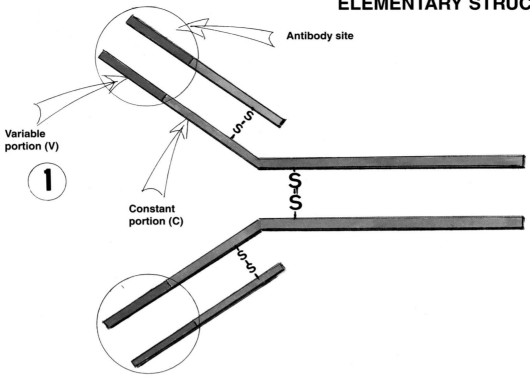

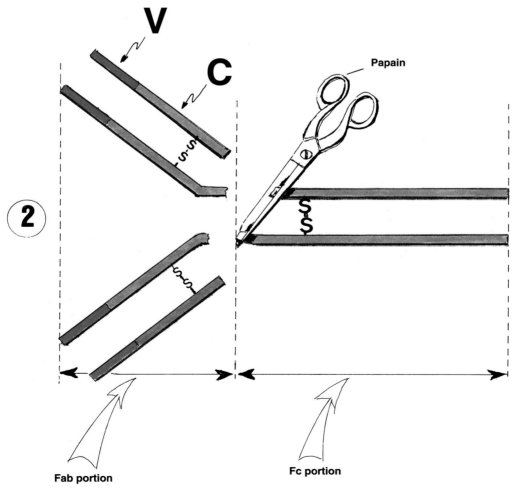

Figure 24

ACTION OF IMMUNOGLOBULINS

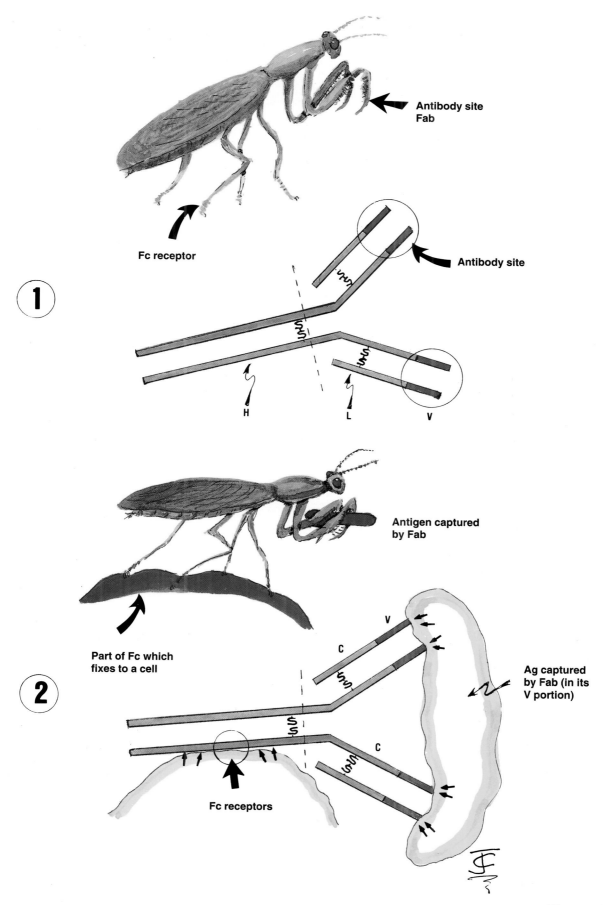

1

Antibody site
Fab

Fc receptor

Antibody site

H   L   V

2

Antigen captured
by Fab

Part of Fc which
fixes to a cell

Fc receptors

V   C   C

Ag captured
by Fab (in its
V portion)

Figure 25

CLASSES OF IMMUNOGLOBULINS

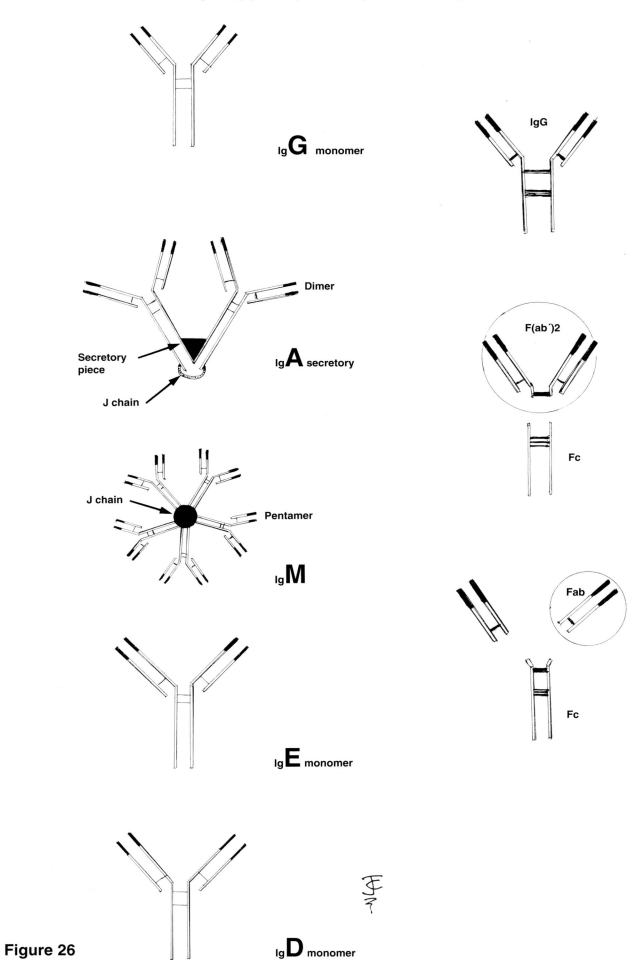

Figure 26

1.9.4 Immunoglobulin Classes

Five classes of Ig are known: IgG, IgA, IgM, IgE, and IgD **(Figure 26)**. Their essential characteristics are as follows:

1. **IgG**: represents 75–80% of the total Ig in man. IgG crosses the placental barrier. Thus, at birth, a baby temporarily carries IgG of its mother, which lasts for 4–6 months.

IgG diffuses into the plasma. It intervenes in infections by means of **opsonization** and it can neutralize **toxins**. IgG appears especially following a secondary immune response, i. e., after a second encounter with antigen. The secretion of IgG is modulated by collaboration between B and T lymphocytes. IgG is strongly opsonizing for macrophages and polymorphonuclears, possessing receptors for the Fc fragment of IgG.

There are four IgG subclasses: **IgG1, IgG2, IgG3**, and **IgG4**, and all of these, except IgG4, have the ability to fix complement.

2. **IgA** represents about 15% of plasma Ig. It is mainly involved in the defense of mucous membranes and probably also in the elimination of certain antigens. This elimination proceeds discretely, without contribution of the "virulent" complement, since IgA does not fix the latter (at least through the classical pathway). Defense of mucous membranes is ensured by secretory IgA. These are dimers. The two monomers forming the dimer are connected by a small **polypeptide J chain**, synthesized by IgA-secreting plasmocytes. Monomeric IgA form plasma IgA, which are eliminated by the liver.

Secretory IgA (IgA-s) are synthesized mainly at the level of the lamina propria by A plasmocytes. (The lamina propria is found in intestinal villi under the mucous membrane.)

There are two subclasses of IgA: **IgA 1** and **IgA 2** (depending on the disulfide bridges between the H and L chains). Secretory IgA resists digestive enzymes due to the **secretory component**. This component is fixed to the dimer and is synthesized in epithelial cells, where it acts at the level of cell membranes as an IgA receptor. This dimeric IgA with its secretory piece attached is transported then to the luminal pole of the cell, i. e., the pole corresponding to the lumen of the organ (e. g., discharge into the intestinal lumen).

The secretory IgA or IgA-s does not opsonize. It fixes antigen via its variable part and forms unabsorbed complexes. By capturing antigens, it prevents bacteria and viruses from adhering to the mucous membrane, thereby preventing their penetration into the organism.

The Fc fragment of IgA does not play any role, probably because it is obstructed by the secretory component.

IgA deficiency is normally encountered in one of 700 individuals, causing in such patients more frequent respiratory or gastrointestinal infections. According to Burnet, IgA serves as "an antiseptic layer of paint on the mucosae". In case of IgA deficiency, IgM can take over. In severe cases, there may be a simultaneous deficiency of both IgA and IgM.

Aside from secretory IgA, monomeric serum IgA might play an important role in defense. Since they do not trigger the "irritable" complement, they eliminate discretely, without inflammatory reaction, certain antigens (especially food antigens) having passed through the mucous membrane despite of the secretory IgA. Thus, they would serve as kind of second line of defense. Serum IgA are synthesized mainly in lymphoid tissues not directly linked to mucous membranes: spleen, bone marrow, and lymphatic ganglions. Their final fate is unknown. In man, they are probably metabolized in the liver.

3. **IgM**: represents about 10% of immunoglobulins. They are pentamers (5 units), the monomeric units being fixed by a J chain. They are also known as **macroglobulins** or **heavy globulins**. IgM are the first to appear in an immune response (primary reaction, **Figure 28**). As it has a short life span, its presence points out to a recent infection (e. g., in toxoplasmosis). Due to its polyvalent structure, IgM can easily produce agglutination and readily fixes complement. Because of its large volume, it remains localized principally in blood. It does not cross the placental barrier and is the first molecule to meet a viral or microbial intruder in a blood vessel.

4. **IgD** is only present in small amounts and does not fix complement. Its role is not well understood. It appears on the surface of lymphocytes before IgM, and its concentration increases in some diseases, such as D myeloma or kwashiorkor.

5. **IgE** is only present in minute amounts in normal individuals. It is a cytophilic Ig, i. e., it fixes to the surface of certain cells, especially mast cells and basophils. Furthermore, it is homocytotropic, i.e, only fixing to cells of the same type. It does not fix complement. IgE occurs predominantly in perivascular tissues where mast cells are localized. **IgEs are responsible for type I allergic reactions**. IgE levels are much higher in patients suffering from type I allergies. The binding of IgE with an antigen specific to this IgE on the mast cell membrane provokes expulsion of mast cell granules **(degranulation)**. The granules contain a large number of mediators.

IgE plays a major role in allergy, but it also appears to intervene in the defense against parasites and perhaps also against cancer cells. A high IgE level in apparently healthy babies is a fairly accurate indicator of later allergic disorders.

IgE levels are particularly elevated in atopic eczema and in intestinal parasitoses. Similarly elevated levels are also found in certain myelomas and in disorders involving a long- or short-term deficiency in T lymphocytes: measles, mononucleosis, Hodgkin's disease, dysglobulinemia, etc. The important role played by specific IgE in type I allergies will be discussed in greater detail later.

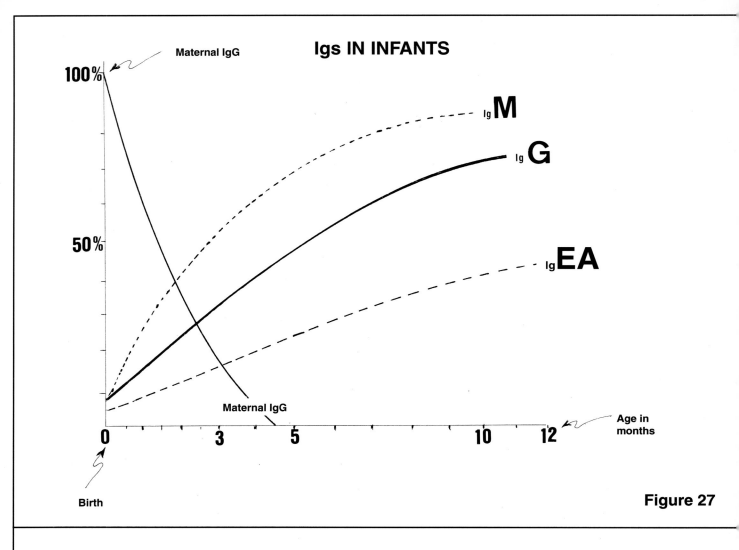

Igs IN INFANTS

Maternal IgG

100%

IgM

IgG

50%

IgEA

Maternal IgG

Age in months

0   3   5   10   12

Birth

Figure 27

IgG AND IgM DURING AN INFECTION

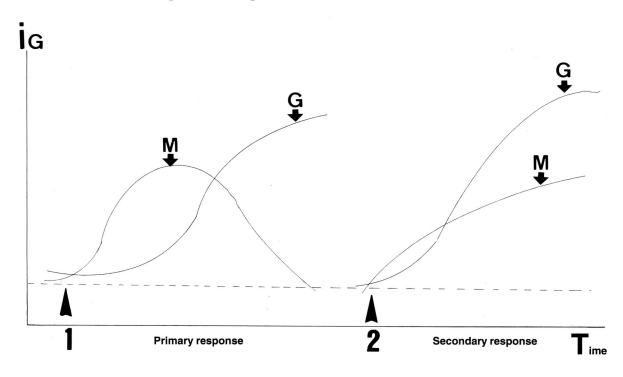

IG

G

M

G

M

1   Primary response   2   Secondary response   Time

Figure 28

1.9.5 Antibodies at birth

The curve in **Figure 27** shows the evolution of serum Ig concentrations in babies, depending on age. At birth (point 0), a baby possesses 100% of his immunoglobulins (IgG) from the mother, but only very little IgA or IgM. The slightest infection, however, increases the IgM level considerably. Mother's Igs are metabolized between the third and fifth month. Towards the sixth month of life, the baby has synthesized about 33% of his IgG, 30% of IgA, and 70% of IgM, the own IgG production not starting until the second month. IgA and IgE are produced last.

One may therefore visualize that if immunoglobulin synthesis is delayed, the infant may pass through a period of **physiological hypogammaglobulinemia**. This arises when the infant has eliminated maternal IgG but has not yet synthesized enough of his own. There occurs, thus, a temporary deficiency with a corresponding transient increased susceptibility to bacterial infections. **Figure 27** shows an approximate picture of the evolution of blood Ig concentration, varying slightly from one individual to another.

1.9.6 IgM and IgG in primary and secondary immune responses

The graph in **Figure 28** shows the evolution of IgM and IgG during infection. During a first infection ❶, antigen stimulation causes IgM to appear first, with IgG appearing a few days later. This is the **primary response.** Detection of specific IgM in blood permits us to suspect a recent infection. If, for example, antitoxoplasmosis or anti-rubella antibodies of the IgM class are found in a patient, a recent primary infection may be diagnosed. In subsequent infections ❷, specific IgG antibodies appear quickly and in large amounts. This is the **secondary response**. Thus, the presence of anti-measles virus or anti-Toxoplasma antibodies of the IgG class signifies an old infection, in contrast to the IgM-type, which points to a recent infection.

REGULATION OF IgE PRODUCTION

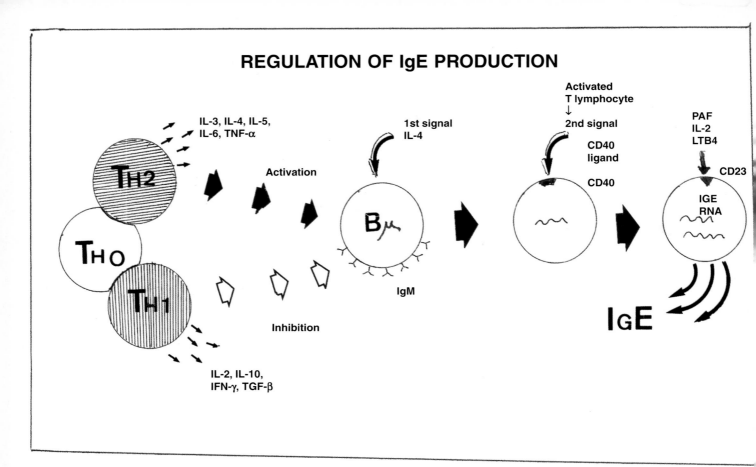

MAIN IgE REGULATORS

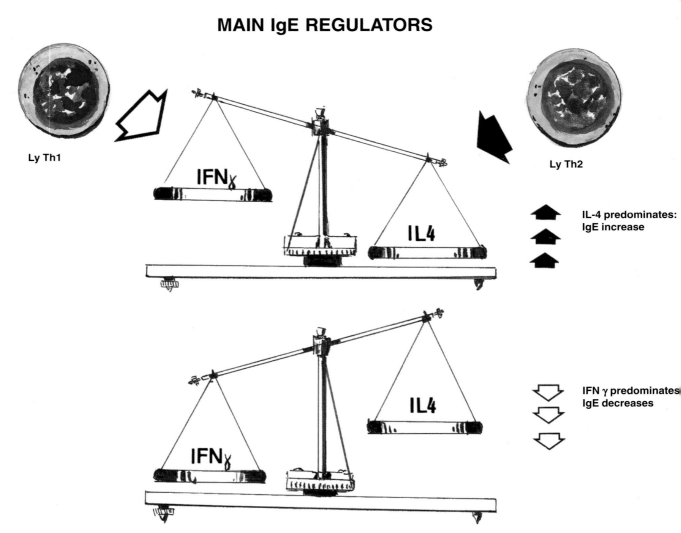

Figure 29

1.9.7 Immunoglobulins E and their Regulation.

In view to their primordial role in most frequent allergic diseases and the special characteristics of their regulation, IgE merits a considerably more thorough discussion. Although anaphylactic reactions of type I and particularly the accompanying skin reactions had been correlated since 1920 with some specific substance in serum enabling passive transfer (Prausnitz-Küstner reaction) and called "reagin," the fifth class of antibodies, immunoglobulin E, was only definitely identified in 1967. The main reason for this enduring mystery is the very low level of IgE in serum, compared to other Ig: normally 100–200 ng IgE/ml, i.e., a remarkable 10,000 times less than IgG!

The production of IgE follows different rules than that of other Ig: maximal IgE production is only achieved by relatively infrequent exposure to very low concentrations of allergens (in the microgram range). In contrast, more frequent contact with allergens favors production of IgG. Some bacteria (Bordetella pertussis, responsible for whooping cough) or chemical adjuvants (aluminum hydroxide) particularly enhance IgE production.

In normal individuals, IgE production is generally suppressed in an efficient manner. However, when the suppressor mechanism is temporarily put out of order, e. g., during some viral infections (rhinovirus, infectious mononucleosis), the encounter of a strong allergen may initiate a prolonged IgE formation. This phenomenon was called "allergic breakthrough," and it explains why some individuals may suddenly become very allergic against some isolated allergens which they tolerated well up to that moment.

This form of allergy and IgE response regulation has to be distinguished from a more general trend to form IgE, as encountered in the atopic syndrome or during some immune deficiencies. In these cases, a permanent alteration of the immunological balance between helper and suppressor T lymphocytes is probably responsible for the elevated IgE level.

In recent years, research has focused on the differentiation of B lymphocytes and the regulation of IgE synthesis **(Figure 29)**. Not yet differentiated B lymphocytes carrying only IgM on their surface (Bμ) will differentiate into IgE-producing cells under the impulse of a first signal provided by IL-4, followed by a second signal which involves a cellular receptor called CD40. The second signal is provided by a molecule called "CD40 ligand," which is expressed on activated T lymphocytes, but also on some other activated cells (e. g., B lymphocytes infected with the Epstein-Barr virus). The result of both signals is the intranuclear expression of two messenger RNAs characteristic for IgE: a short germ-line IgE mRNA and a long IgE mRNA coding for the IgE molecule. Activated B lymphocytes switching to IgE production also express a receptor with low affinity for IgE **(FcεRII)**, known under the name of CD23. The expression of this receptor is likewise under the influence of various cytokines, such as IL-2 and IL-4 or various inflammatory mediators, such as LTB4 and PAF. In this scheme, cytokines produced by helper T lymphocytes of the Th2 class favor IgE production while some lymphokines produced by Th1 lymphocytes, particularly IFN γ and TGF β, strongly inhibit the expression of IgE mRNAs.

IMMUNISATION BY AN Ag CARRYING VARIOUS EPITOPES

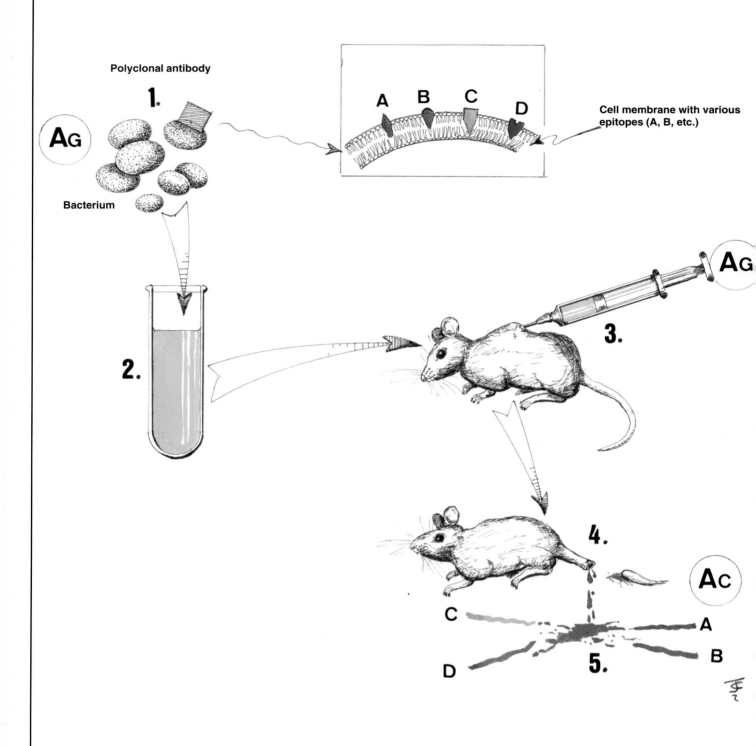

Polyclonal antibody

1.

Ag

Bacterium

A B C D

Cell membrane with various epitopes (A, B, etc.)

2.

3.

Ag

4.

Ac

C

A

D

B

5.

Figure 30

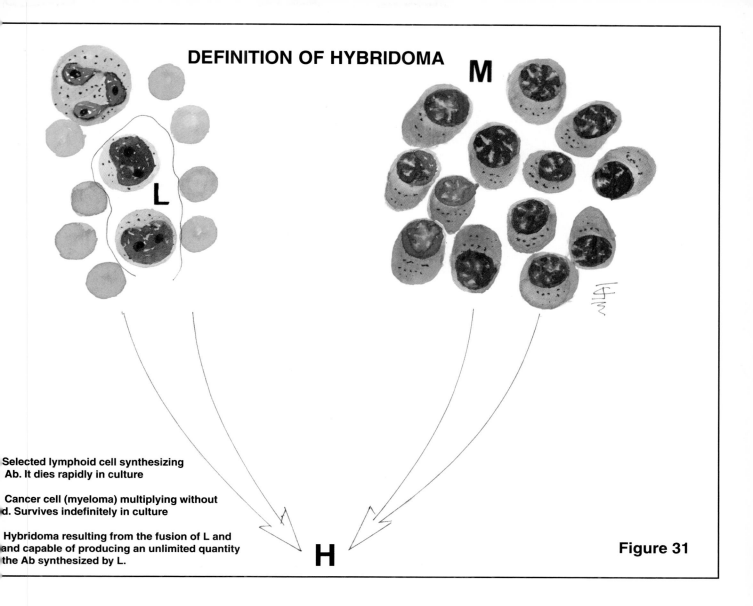

DEFINITION OF HYBRIDOMA

L

M

H

Selected lymphoid cell synthesizing Ab. It dies rapidly in culture

Cancer cell (myeloma) multiplying without d. Survives indefinitely in culture

Hybridoma resulting from the fusion of L and and capable of producing an unlimited quantity the Ab synthesized by L.

Figure 31

1.10 Monoclonal Antibodies (MAb) – Chimeric Antibodies and Repertoire Cloning

1.10.1 Definitions

The ability to produce MAb has been a major advance in immunology. Its principle is illustrated in **Figure 31**.

What is a MAb? It is an antibody **specific to only one antigenic determinant or epitope**. An antigen is known to be a chemical structure, such as a protein, or a particulate element, such as a bacterium, red blood cell, parasite, etc. which in fact encompasses numerous antigenic sites or so called antigenic determinants **(Figure 30)**.

Figure 30: Taking the example of bacteria. A drawing of the bacterial cell wall shows its lipoprotein double layer with membrane proteins or polysaccharides carrying their various epitopes A, B, C, D, ❶. In reality, there may be a huge number of such epitopes, even thousands.

If this antigen in suspension ❷ is injected into a mouse ❸, the mouse will synthesize a mixture of specific antibodies (polyclonal antibodies) against each determinant: anti-A, anti-B, anti-C and anti-D ❹ and so on. Each color in ❹ represents a specific circulating antibody directed against a single determinant. As an example, cancer cells carry determinants on their membrane which are difficult to identify with precision and to distinguish from determinants on membranes of normal cells in the same tissue. MAb, however, are specific to each separate determinant, allowing us to single out determinants (or membrane Ag) of cancer cells from those of other cells. In reality, as will be shown, things are not quite that simple.

The problem is to isolate monoclonal antibodies specific to the determinant or the determinants in question, and to produce them in large quantities.

55

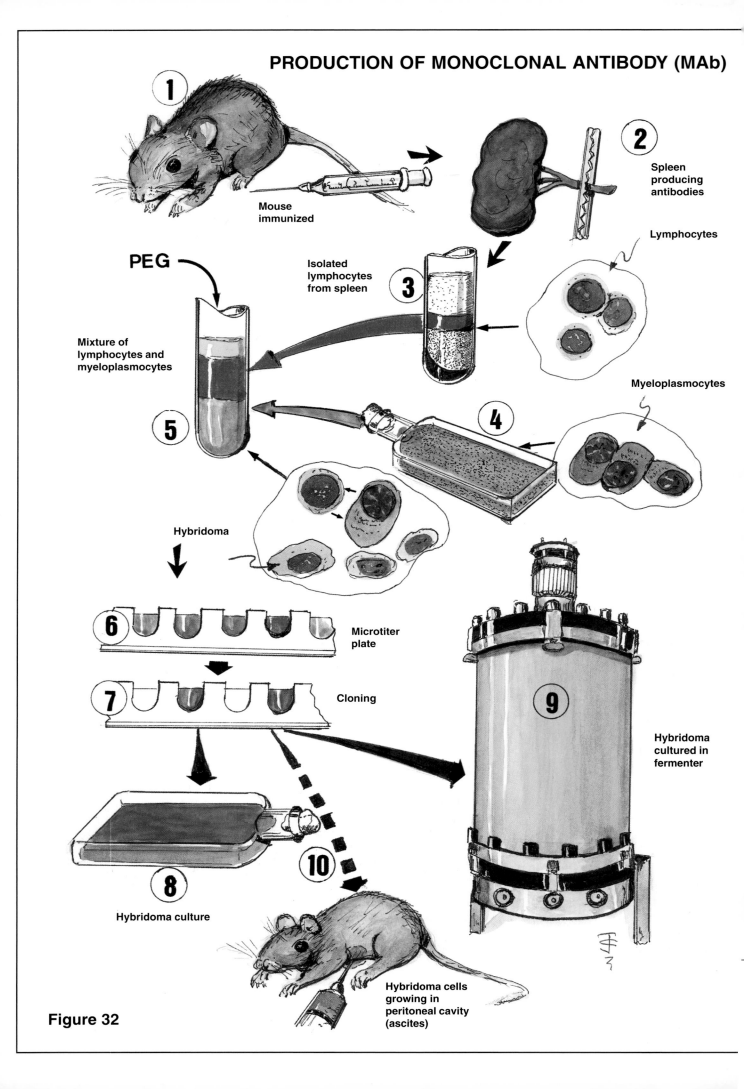

PRODUCTION OF MONOCLONAL ANTIBODY (MAb)

1 — Mouse immunized

2 — Spleen producing antibodies

Lymphocytes

Isolated lymphocytes from spleen

3

PEG

Mixture of lymphocytes and myeloplasmocytes

5

Myeloplasmocytes

4

Hybridoma

6 — Microtiter plate

7 — Cloning

9 — Hybridoma cultured in fermenter

8 — Hybridoma culture

10 — Hybridoma cells growing in peritoneal cavity (ascites)

Figure 32

1.10.2 Production of monoclonal antibodies (MAb)

To understand the principle underlying the production of monoclonal antibodies, it must be recalled that antibody-secreting B lymphocytes do not survive in culture. Some tumor cells, however, may survive indefinitely under culture conditions.

Figure 31: The principle of producing monoclonal antibodies consists of combining within a single cell the "immortality" of a tumor cell and the specific antibody production capacity of a B lymphocyte. The tumor cell acts as motor, and the B lymphocyte as manufacturer of Ig. Fusion of these two cells results in a single cell, called a **hybridoma** (H). Each hybridoma synthesizes one single type of specific antibody, i. e., directed against only one antigenic determinant. Hybridoma technology permits theoretically production of an unlimited number of wanted MAbs.

Figure 32 shows the production process of MAbs:

In ❶, a mouse is immunized with an antigen suspension. Although this antigen carries several determinants, only one of them is of interest to us. Our aim will be to isolate the required antibody directed against one single determinant, separate it, and then produce it in large amounts.

In ❷, after due time, the mouse will have produced a whole range of antibodies which are secreted mainly by lymphoid organs such as spleen and lymph nodes. At this point, we remove the spleen.

In ❸, the isolated spleen is ground up, filtered and mixed with a sterile culture medium. The mixture is centrifuged, yielding the following layers: red blood cells, culture medium, and a characteristic ring of lymphoid cells (shown in red in the diagram) which is of interest to us.

In ❹, a culture of tumoral plasmocytes (in blue) originating from a myeloma is shown. These are myeloma cells (myeloplasmocytes).

In ❺, tumoral and lymphoid cells are mixed and incubated.

A polyethylene glycol mixture (PEG) is then added to facilitate fusion of the lymphoid cells with the myeloplasmocytes. It is at this stage that the first major problem arises, as only a limited number of fused cells or hybridomas is obtained. Among non-fused cells, lymphocytes die spontaneously, whereas myeloplasmocytes develop to the point of even taking over the whole culture. Therefore, it is important to remove them beforehand. This is achieved by treating the myeloplasmocytes with a special culture medium (HAT) before fusion. In such a medium, only fused cells will continue to grow. Many technical details involved in this process are beyond the scope of this publication.

In ❻, hybridomas are separated (by extreme dilution) and placed in microplaque wells. They are then investigated for antibody production, and the antibodies produced are identified by analysis of culture supernatants.

In ❼, the hybridomas producing the antibodies of interest to us are selected and deposited in a new well where they may be left to proliferate. This is known as **cloning**.

In ❽, clones are then either cultured in large amounts in a suitable medium or injected into the peritoneum of a histocompatible mouse ❿. A large amount of MAb is obtained in this way. Nowadays, mass production of such antibodies may be entirely achieved in vitro by using techniques analogous to fermentation ❾, avoiding in this way a cruel method involving experimental animals.

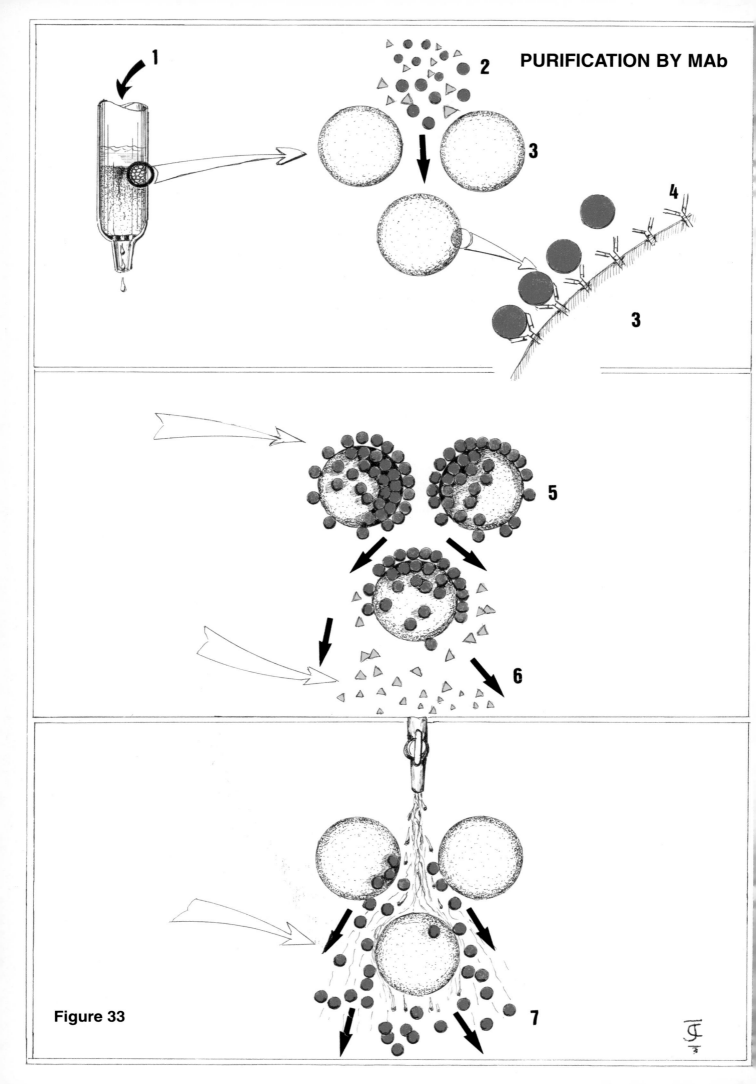

PURIFICATION BY MAb

Figure 33

1.10.3 Value of monoclonal antibodies – Examples of use

The discovery of MAb has been the basis of a considerable number of studies concerning a variety of fields: biochemistry, microbiology, oncology, pregnancy tests, forensic medicine, vaccines, toxicology, physiology, etc.

We can only very briefly review the wide range of applications for Mab which have been developed, to provide some flavor of the essential principles, difficulties and expectations involved.

MAb are specific to a single epitope forming part of an often complex antigen. The epitope permits us to identify, isolate or separate an antigen from a mixture. **Figures 33** and **34** illustrate this process, the principle of which is applied to numerous analyses and purifications.

In **Figure 33,** the mixture for analysis is introduced into a suitable tube ❶. For simplification the drawing here only shows two epitopes, one represented by red circles and the other by yellow triangles ❷. A MAb ❹ fixed to beads ❸ is directed against the "red circled" epitope. During passage of the solution containing the antigen mixture, the MAb "catches" ❺ the red circles, allowing the yellow triangles to pass ❻. Finally, the "red circled" epitopes are recovered by washing. An extremely pure product is thus obtained.

The discovery of Mab allowed us to make great progress in increasing the specificity of diagnostic tests. In **Figure 34** the "solid" phase is represented by the walls of a tube. The MAb (green) is fixed to the wall of the tube ❶. The solution or the biological fluid (e. g., serum) containing antigen to be detected (e. g., hormone, IgE antibody, etc.) (yellow) is added; it carries an epitope recognized by the fixed MAb ❷. In order to make visible the complex that is formed by adding ❶ and ❷ together, another MAb directed against another epitope of the antigen to be detected is used (this is the so called "sandwich" technique). This second antibody, called a revealing antibody, may be either labeled by a radioactive atom ❸ (in red) according to the RIA technique, or by an enzyme ❹ (in blue), according to the ELISA technique.

In cytology and hematology, MAbs enable us to identify, classify, and isolate cell lines, to specify a stage of differen-tiation, to locate abnormal cells, and to follow the course of a disease during treatment. Numerous MAbs are commercially available which recognize surface antigens of hematopoietic cells. For example CD3 for T lymphocytes (OKT3), CD4 (OKT4) to label Th lymphocytes, and CD8 (OKT8) for cytotoxic and Ts lymphocytes, etc.

Leukaemic cells may be identified in a cell suspension. **Figure 35** shows in **A** the microscopic appearance of leukaemic blood. It is virtually impossible to differentiate and to count the pathological cells under the microscope. In **B**, these cells have been marked with an MAb combined with a fluorescent dye (immunofluorescence). The leukemic cells can be separated from normal cells by flow cytometry (FACS) sorting. For example, this method is used to "purge" bone marrow of its pathological cells before a graft. In some forms of leukemia, the patient's own bone marrow is removed and stored before aggressive immunosuppressive treatment. After treatment, the patient is reinjected with his own bone marrow, which has been purged of its leukemic cells.

If a **graft versus host reaction** (GVH) is expected, T cells of the graft may be removed thanks to MAb anti-CD3 (OKT3). At present, the majority of such patients are treated with cyclosporin. In the field of transplantation, MAbs permit typing for HLA groups in a more precise manner. In cancer, it is known that metastases are mainly responsible for the patient's death. Therefore it is important to detect them early in order to attempt their elimination. Using classical techniques, only metastases of more than 0.5 cm in diameter may be demonstrated. One of the new methods made possible by MAbs is immunoscintigraphy.

The principle of **immunoscintigraphy** consists in injecting into a vein some MAb labeled by a radioactive isotope and specific to antigens related to the tumor, locating it when it has fixed to tumor cells. Use of polyclonal antibodies with carcino-embryonic antigen (CEA) and α-fetoprotein was already known.

Immunoscintigraphy is performed by various sophisticated radiotomographic techniques. In practice, however, only about 0.1% of the injected MAb fixes to the tumor. One of the major problems, moreover, is the tissular "background noise," i. e., radioisotopic emission due to non-specific binding of the injected MAb.

IMMUNOLOGICAL DIAGNOSIS WITH AcM

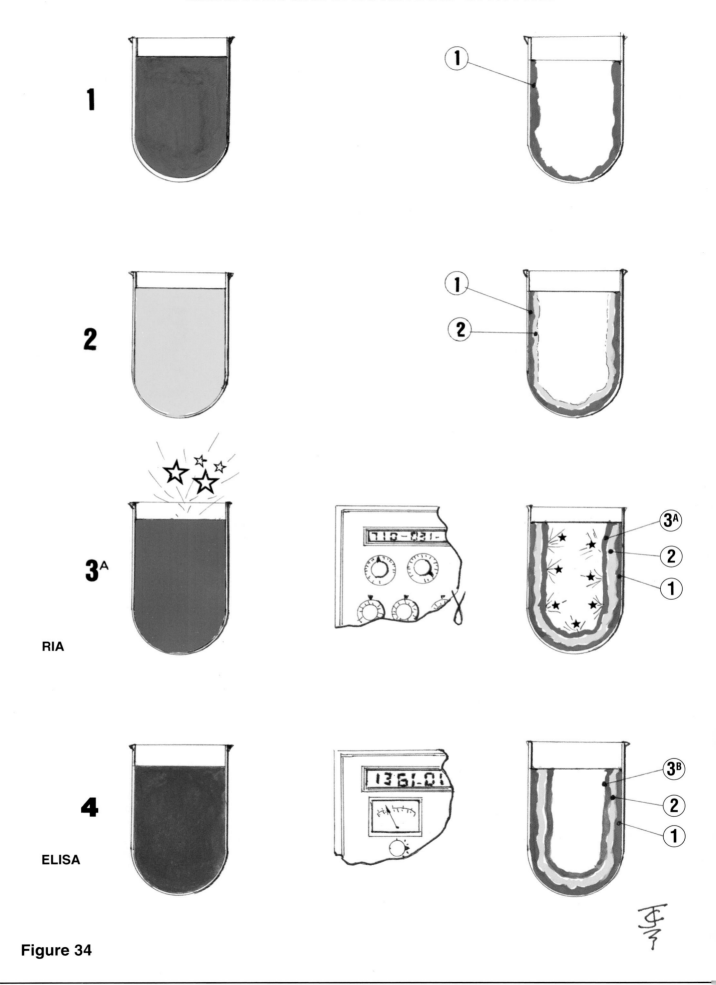

Figure 34

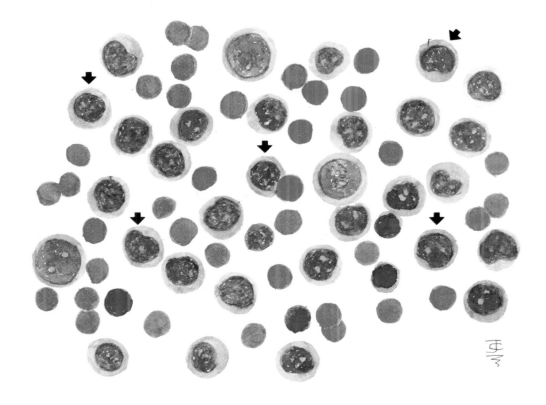

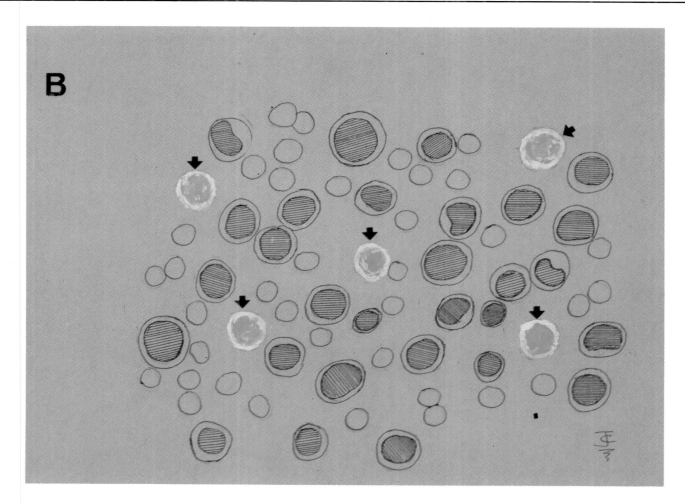

Figure 35

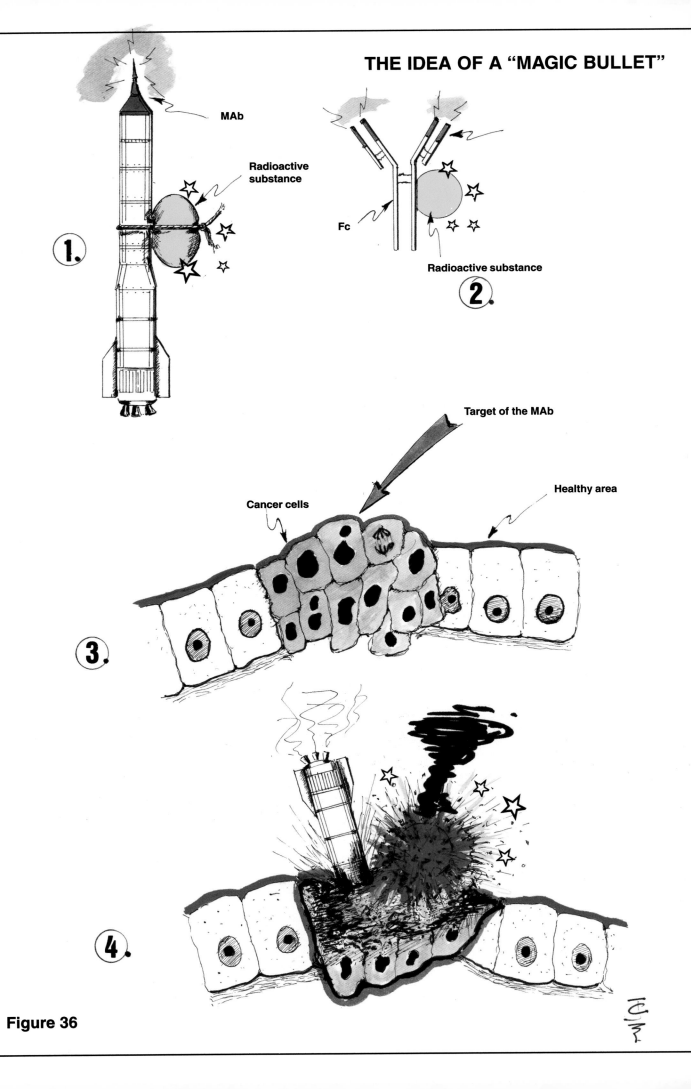

THE IDEA OF A "MAGIC BULLET"

Figure 36

1.10.4 The researchers' dreams

By the discovery of MAbs, researchers became very hopeful that specific antibodies might be produced for each type of tumor and could be used as vectors directed exclusively at the tumor. Combined with an isotope, it would then allow the tumor to be located exactly by scintigraphy (+ scanner) and its volume to be assessed.

It was also hoped that MAb could be used as vector for transporting a toxin (e. g., ricin) or a radioactive substance, or even for attracting complement to destroy cancer cells, sparing the normal tissue around the tumor. This was the

"magic bullet." It was a dream! **(Figs. 36–37)**, but researchers were soon to be disappointed: the situation "in vitro" is not the same as "in vivo." **The majority of tumors do not express tumor specific antigens on their surfaces**. In addition, their poor vascularization prevents diffusion of MAbs (IgG diffuses better than IgM, for example).

Figure 36: The "magic bullet": MAb was assumed to be specific to the Ag of the cancer (in green). It is used to carry a radioactive substance, fixed to the Fc part of the MAb ❷, to target the cancer ❸ and thus to destroy it ❹.

THE RESEARCHER'S DREAM

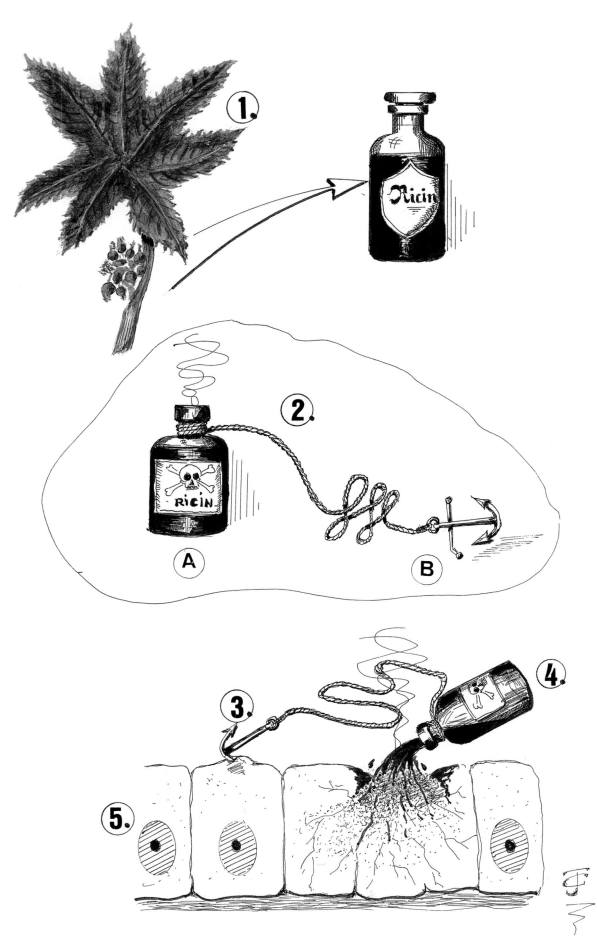

Figure 37

Figure 37: Another researcher's dream: to couple a MAb specific to a cancer cell to a toxin. Use of castor oil toxin ❶ coupled to a MAb ❷, enabling to target the conjugate ❸ ❹ against the tumor cells to be destroyed ❺. **(A)** denotes the toxic active part of castor oil. **(B)** shows the MAb molecule that anchors castor oil in the tissues.

However, the realization of these dreams has met with many difficulties. Part of the MAb is captured non-specifically by macrophages, provoking what is known as "background noise," which considerably disturbs the scintigraphic images. The patient can also develop reactions against the MAb itself or against foreign proteins contaminating the MAb, because MAbs are produced in animal or in cell cultures and may in this process be contaminated by various proteins. Part of the MAb may be captured by circulating tumor antigens, released by necrotic tumor cells detached from the tumor. Furthermore, the affinity of MAbs is often low. All these considerations account for the fact that reality is often less promising than theory.

Unfortunately, further details concerning MAb techniques, although fascinating and practical, are beyond the frame of this volume.

CHIMERIC ANTIBODIES

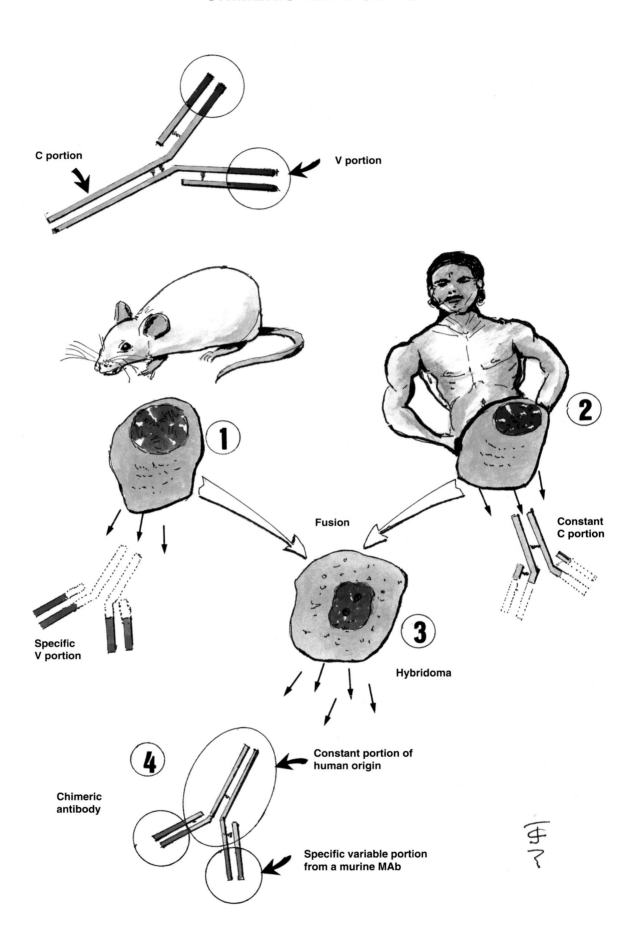

C portion

V portion

Fusion

Specific
V portion

Constant
C portion

Hybridoma

Constant portion of
human origin

Chimeric
antibody

Specific variable portion
from a murine MAb

Figure 38A

1.10.5 Chimeric antibodies and repertoire cloning

Molecular biological techniques now allow us to create molecules which are called "chimeric," so named in an analogy with the exotic animals of mythology which were composed of parts belonging to diverse animal species.

Creation of chimera may happen in several ways, e. g.:
a) fusion of cells producing various antibody fragments (e. g., hybridomas between mouse and human B cells) **(Figure 38 A)**
b) in vitro assembly of genes or of DNA fragments, followed by their multiplication through **PCR** (Polymerase Chain Reaction), transcription to RNA and expression as protein by an appropriate vector (e. g., Escherichia coli) **(Figure 38 B)**. This procedure is described in more detail in Chapter 4.1 Recombinant allergens.

Figure 38 A. With the use of these chimeric antibodies, it is therefore possible to produce very interesting antibodies which have components from both mouse and man. In these cases, the variable portions of antibodies determining their specificity (CDR: complementarity Determining Region) stem from one highly defined murine monoclonal antibody ❶, while the constant part of the immunoglobulin molecule stems from a human source ❷. In this way ❸, it is possible to obtain chimeric antibodies ❹ of very high affinity, possibly even against antigens which may not be injected in man. Such hybrid antibodies are very similar to native human antibodies and will not be readily rejected, as occurs for murine antibodies repeatedly injected in man.

The genetic **repertoire** may be defined as the total collection of genes possessed by an individual, which enable him to produce a wide array of antibodies of very different specificities and affinities. The procedure of cloning the repertoire's immunoglobulins **("repertoire cloning")** occurs entirely in vitro and permits us indeed to produce virtually any kind of antibody without involving an antibody-producing animal.

PRINCIPLE OF REPERTOIRE CLONING OF SPECIFIC IMMUNOGLOBULINS

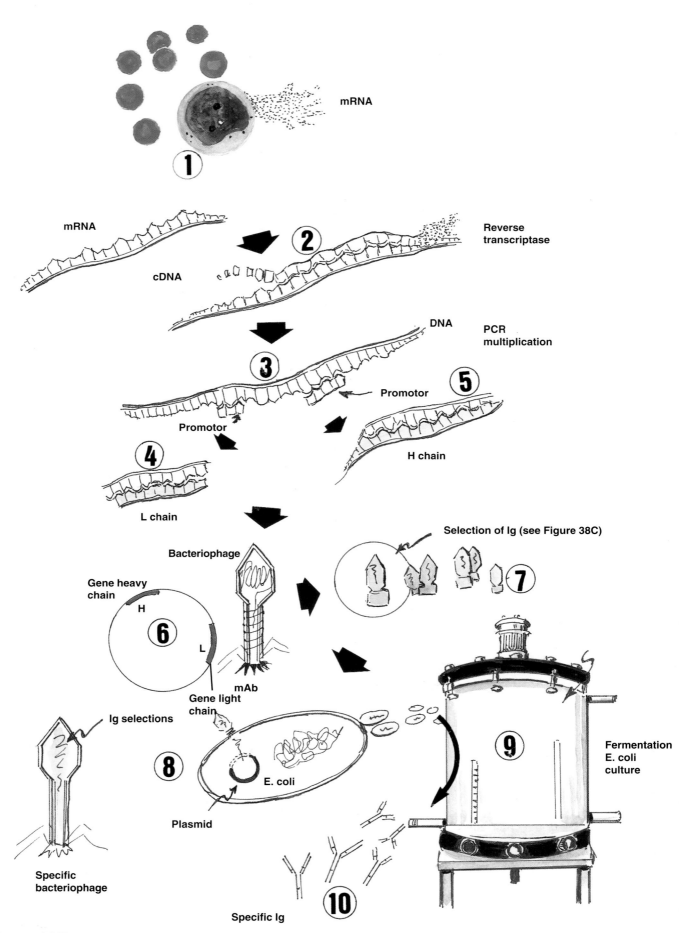

Figure 38B

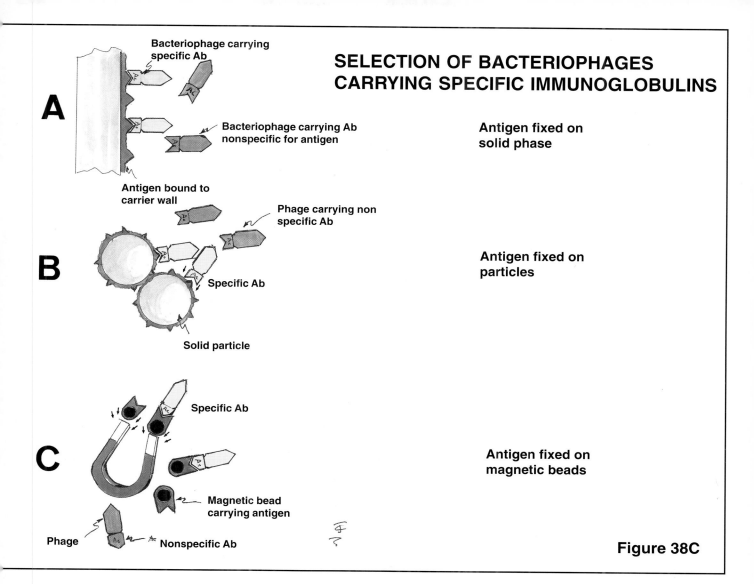

SELECTION OF BACTERIOPHAGES CARRYING SPECIFIC IMMUNOGLOBULINS

A

Bacteriophage carrying specific Ab

Bacteriophage carrying Ab nonspecific for antigen

Antigen bound to carrier wall

Antigen fixed on solid phase

B

Phage carrying non specific Ab

Specific Ab

Solid particle

Antigen fixed on particles

C

Specific Ab

Magnetic bead carrying antigen

Phage Nonspecific Ab

Antigen fixed on magnetic beads

Figure 38C

Figure 38 B. At the beginning of this process, the total messenger RNA (mRNA) of human B lymphocytes is extracted from peripheral blood ❶. Out of this mRNA, corresponding DNA chains are deducted and synthesized (transcription) ❷ by means of the enzyme "reverse transcriptase." From this very complex mixture of genes and DNA chains, it becomes possible for the DNA chains to multiply in a very selective manner, corresponding to heavy (H) and light (L) immunoglobulin chains. This selection is effected by defined **promoters** ("primers") enabling the multiplication of selected DNA chains through a procedure called **PCR (Polymerase Chain reaction)** ❸.

In order to enable the selection of not only the ensemble of immunoglobulins, but also of those specific for a given antigen ❹ and ❺, genes multiplied by PCR are introduced in the genome of a bacteriophage, e.g., of type p Comb 3 ❻. This bacteriophage recombines the genes of H and L chains and expresses one single reconstituted immunoglobulin molecule on the wall of the bacteriophage.

Although in the beginning these bacteriophages represent a mixture of immunoglobulins with all specificities included in the repertoire, putting them in contact with antigen enables us to select those bacteriophages carrying immunoglobulins specific for the chosen antigen. Selection may occur by various immunoadsorption techniques, as described in more detail in **Figure 38 C.** The specifically selected bacteriophages are allowed to multiply in culture and are further purified by several cycles of adhesion to antigen (procedure of "panning"), followed by multiplication.

Finally, when only bacteriophages strictly specific to the antigen are left, their immunoglobulin genes are introduced into an appropriate vector, **Figure 38B** ❽ (e. g., Escherichia coli, yeast, cells), which when cultured in a fermenter ❾ will produce corresponding proteins in large amounts ❿. They are human antibodies in this case entirely corresponding or very similar to natural antibodies.

Although this technology is still in its beginning, it has already permitted the production of human antibodies which are potentially usable in therapy, such as anti-tetanus or anti-Rhesus antibodies for the prevention of fetal erythroblastosis. In the near future, an industrial application might be developed to revolutionize immunoglobulin therapy, which so far has been based on blood donations and plasma fractionation.

COMPLEMENT

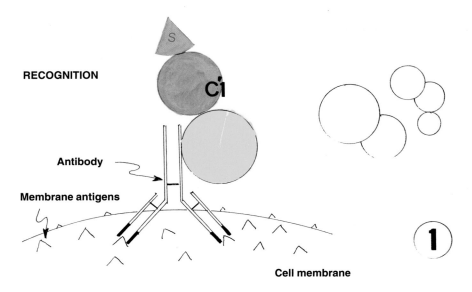

RECOGNITION

Antibody

Membrane antigens

Cell membrane

①

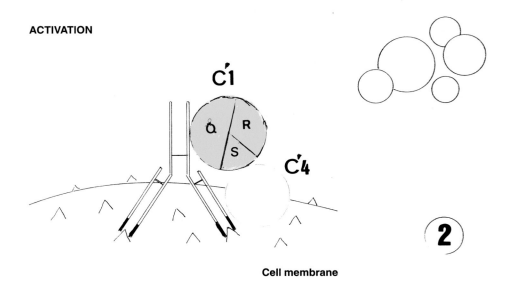

ACTIVATION

Cell membrane

②

Figure 39

1.11 Complement

Complement or more accurately, the **complement system,** consists of a set of 9 pro-enzymes, present in a non-active form in blood **(Figures 39–40)**. These are not surprisingly called C1, C2, C3, C4, C5, C6, C7, C8 and C9. These molecules have molecular weights which range from 79,000 to 400,000 daltons. Their serum concentrations are remarkably variable from the one to the other: C3 is the most abundant, with 1300 µg/ml. In contrast, C6, C7, C8 and C9 are the least abundant, with about 1 µg/ml. C1 consists of three molecules C1q, C1r, and C1s, which are held together by a calcium ion, with about 50 µg/ml for each component

The assembled C1 has six fixation sites. The molecular reactions of complement are very complex and belong to a highly specialized separate field.

The complement system plays a major role in our defense and inflammatory mechanisms. It may intervene by an alternate pathway as soon as an antigen penetrates the organism, well before other mechanisms have had time to mobilize. Together with mechanical defenses, complement is one of our **first lines of defense. It also considerably amplifies certain specific immune mechanisms,** either beneficially or pathologically (e. g., in Arthus phenomenon).

The complement reaction proceeds in a cascading or sequential manner, as in blood coagulation. The first activated element works on the next element and so on, always in the same order: C1, C4, C2, C3, C5, C6, C7, C8, and C9 (however, the order in which these pro-enzymes were named was based on the chronology of their discovery and not on this reaction sequence). **Such a cascade reaction is called "complement fixation."**

The organism possesses inhibitors acting at various stages by modulating and preventing possibly violent and uncontrolled reactions that could be catastrophic.

The complement system reaction may be triggered by many substances, including endotoxin, immune complexes, Fc fragments of IgG1, 2, and 3, IgM, etc. The whole system operates via mechanisms which are still poorly understood, probably involving modifications of their stereochemical structures.

There are two pathways for complement activation:
1. **The "classical" route:** the nine components are activated in sequence, starting with C1.
2. **The "alternate" route:** components C1, C4, and C2 are by-passed and the reaction begins directly with C3. This mechanism is triggered by non-immunological stimuli, such as proteases, endotoxins, plasmin, etc.

This is the pathway which intervenes early in a defense action, before the appearance of antibodies.

Figures 39–40 are only rough diagrams of the sequence, since it is not really possible to draw a reasonable design of such complex physicochemical reactions.

Three phases are distinguished in the reaction: a) recognition, b) activation, and c) attack on cell membrane.
a) **Recognition (Figure 39):** ❶ Ig recognizes an antigenic determinant and fixes to it with its Fab part. The first component of complement, C1 (yellow circle), fixes on the Fc part of the Ig and becomes an active enzyme.
b) **Activation:** ❷ C1 is seen to be composed of three sub-units C1q, C1r and C1s. It is attached via the C1q component to the Fc part of Ig. At this point the C1 site is free and fixes C4 on the cell membrane. This combination must be instantaneous or it does not take place. In **Figure 40**, ❸, C4 fixes C2 and forms a C4-C2 complex called **C3 convertase.** C2 may release a polypeptide which, if not quickly neutralized, may provoke angioneurotic edema (also called Quincke's edema). Some people lack the C1 inhibitor normally required to neutralize the reaction of C1–C2 activation, and as a result they suffer from congenital or familial angioneurotic edema.

COMPLEMENT ACTIVATION

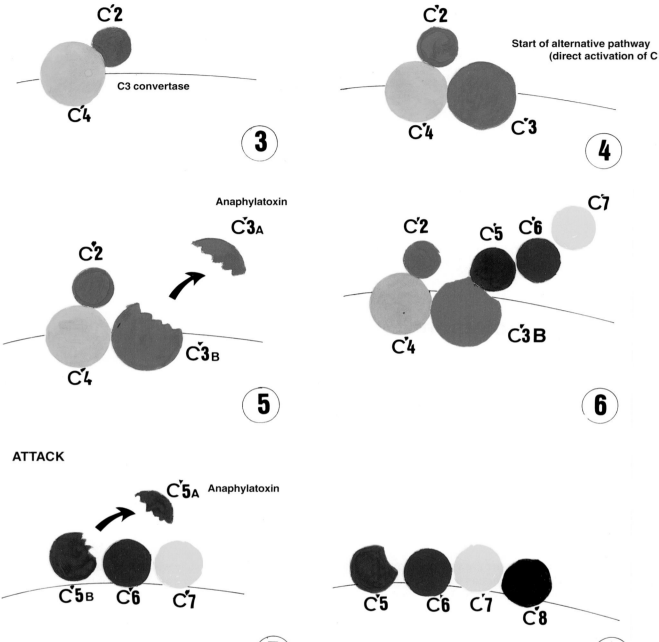

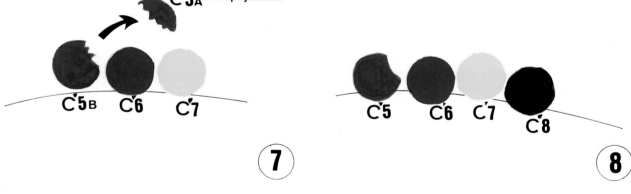

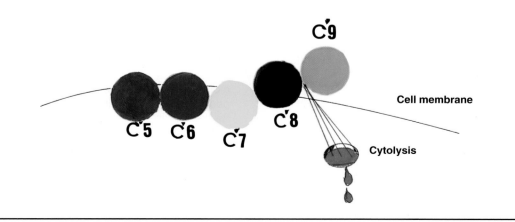

Figure 40

By now, thousands of molecules have been activated, due to the work of C1 (**Figure 40** – ❹ and ❺). There is **amplification**.

C4 and C2 will in turn activate component C3, which itself covers cell membranes. This phenomenon stops immediately if the contacts do not happen very quickly (a nice example of various built-in safety measures). **C3 is the major component involved here.** Several C3 molecules are activated and then C3 splits into **C3a** (4%) and **C3b** (96%). **C3a is an anaphylatoxin capable of degranulating mast cells,** provoking vasodilation, and acting as a **chemotactic factor** for neutrophils, attracting them to the site of an immune reaction.

In ❻, C3b (not shown in the drawing) fixes on the cell membrane **(immunoadherence)** in large amounts and has an **opsonizing effect** on Ag-Ab complexes.

c) **Cell membrane attack:** This consists first of the fixation of C5, C6, and C7. In ❼, C5 releases the polypeptide C5a, which is also an **anaphylatoxin** and a **chemotactic factor**. In ❽, the fragment C5b fixes C6, C7 and C8. In ❾, C8 and C9 are finally activated with the ensuing immune **cytolysis** (perforation of cell membrane) and **hemolysis** (when the perforated membrane is that of an erythrocyte).

To **summarize**, the complement system and its complex mechanisms operate in the following manner:

1. Release of **anaphylatoxins**, which may degranulate mast cells and thereby release powerful mediators;
2. Release of **chemotactic factor**s attracting neutrophils and eosinophils to the site of the immune reaction
3. Opsonization by **means of C3b** fixing to membrane receptors of certain cells. Opsonization permits recognition by phagocytotic cells.
4. Promotion of **cell lysis** (microbes and viruses).

THE FOUR TYPES OF IMMUNO-ALLERGIC REACTIONS (after GELL & COOMBS

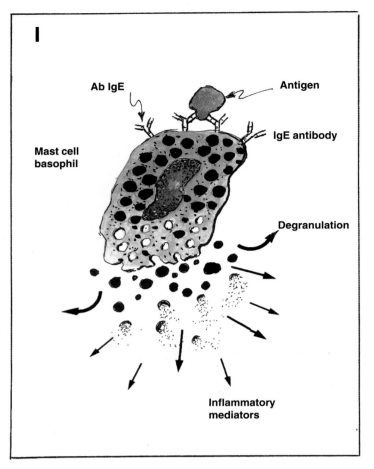

I

Ab IgE

Antigen

IgE antibody

Mast cell
basophil

Degranulation

Inflammatory
mediators

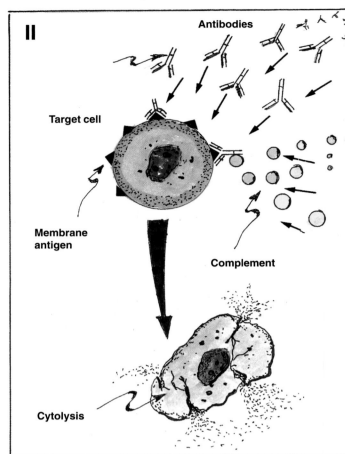

II

Antibodies

Target cell

Membrane
antigen

Complement

Cytolysis

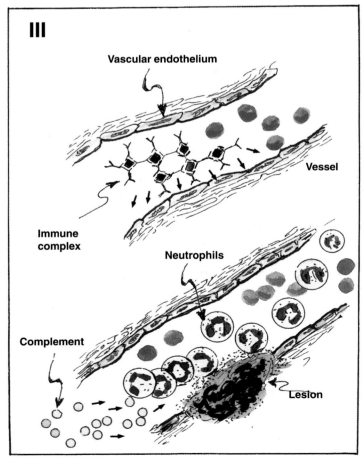

III

Vascular endothelium

Vessel

Immune
complex

Neutrophils

Complement

Lesion

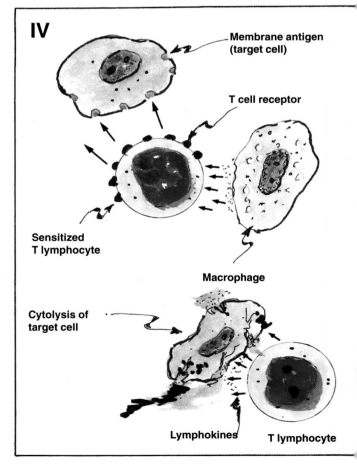

IV

Membrane antigen
(target cell)

T cell receptor

Sensitized
T lymphocyte

Macrophage

Cytolysis of
target cell

Lymphokines

T lymphocyte

Figure 41

1.12 The Four Basic Types of Immuno-allergic Reactions

1.12.1 Generalities

More than 30 years ago, Coombs and Gell ingeniously classified immune reactions into four basic types. Since then, our knowledge has been extended and the now frequent overlaps between the different types should be stressed. Nonetheless this classification is still a very valuable concept for teaching purposes. Physiopathological reality, however, is frequently more complex.

The **four immuno-allergic types according to Gell and Coombs are (Figure 41)**:

- **Type I: anaphylactic reaction ❶**. The antibody fixes onto specific cells: tissue mast cells and basophils in circulating blood. This antibody is called cytotropic or anaphylactic. The antigen reacts with the antibody fixed on the target cell. The antigen-antibody combination on the cell surface triggers release of powerful mediators by the target cells, mast cells and basophils. These are responsible for allergic reactions appearing very fast after antigen-antibody contact, hence the name **"immediate type allergy"** given to type I reactions. The antibodies are mainly IgE and, in some animal species are a subclass of IgG (sometimes called **IgG-STS** for "Short-Term Sensitizing Antibodies").
- **Type II: cytotoxic reaction ❷**. In this case antibody (IgG or IgM) reacts with the antigen fixed to the cell wall of the target cell, especially blood cells. The antigen may be a complete antigen or a hapten. The antigen-antibody reaction by itself does not damage the target cell but may permit intervention of a macrophage. If complement intervenes, reactions are greatly amplified and may lead to cytolysis.
- **Type III: immune complex reaction ❸**. Here the antigen-antibody reaction creates circulating immune complexes, which are deposited in vascular walls or in renal glomeruli. The antibodies involved are IgG or IgM. The immune complexes fix the complement. When the reaction is localized, a violent local response occurs, known as **Arthus phenomenon**, accompanied by thrombosis and hemorrhage. When the reaction is generalized, it is referred to as **"serum-like sickness."** The reaction usually appears a few hours after contact with antigen. This is why it is known as **"semi-delayed allergic reaction."** (Serum sickness used to appear after a massive injection of antitoxin horse serum in diphtheria or tetanus.)
- **Type IV or cell-mediated reaction** (hypersensitivity) ❹. In this type of reaction, the cause is not antibodies circulating in the serum. The reaction starts by an interaction between antigen and specifically sensitized T lymphocytes. These lymphocytes release soluble mediators exerting multiple effects. The reaction develops slowly, over 24 to 48 hours. The process is known as **"delayed type-allergy/hypersensitivity"** or, in comparison, as **"tuberculin-type hypersensitivity,"** because the tuberculin test is typical of type IV reaction.

In autoimmune diseases, Types II, III, and IV may intervene alone or in combination.

The various types of allergic reactions will now be presented in detail.

TYPE I ALLERGY

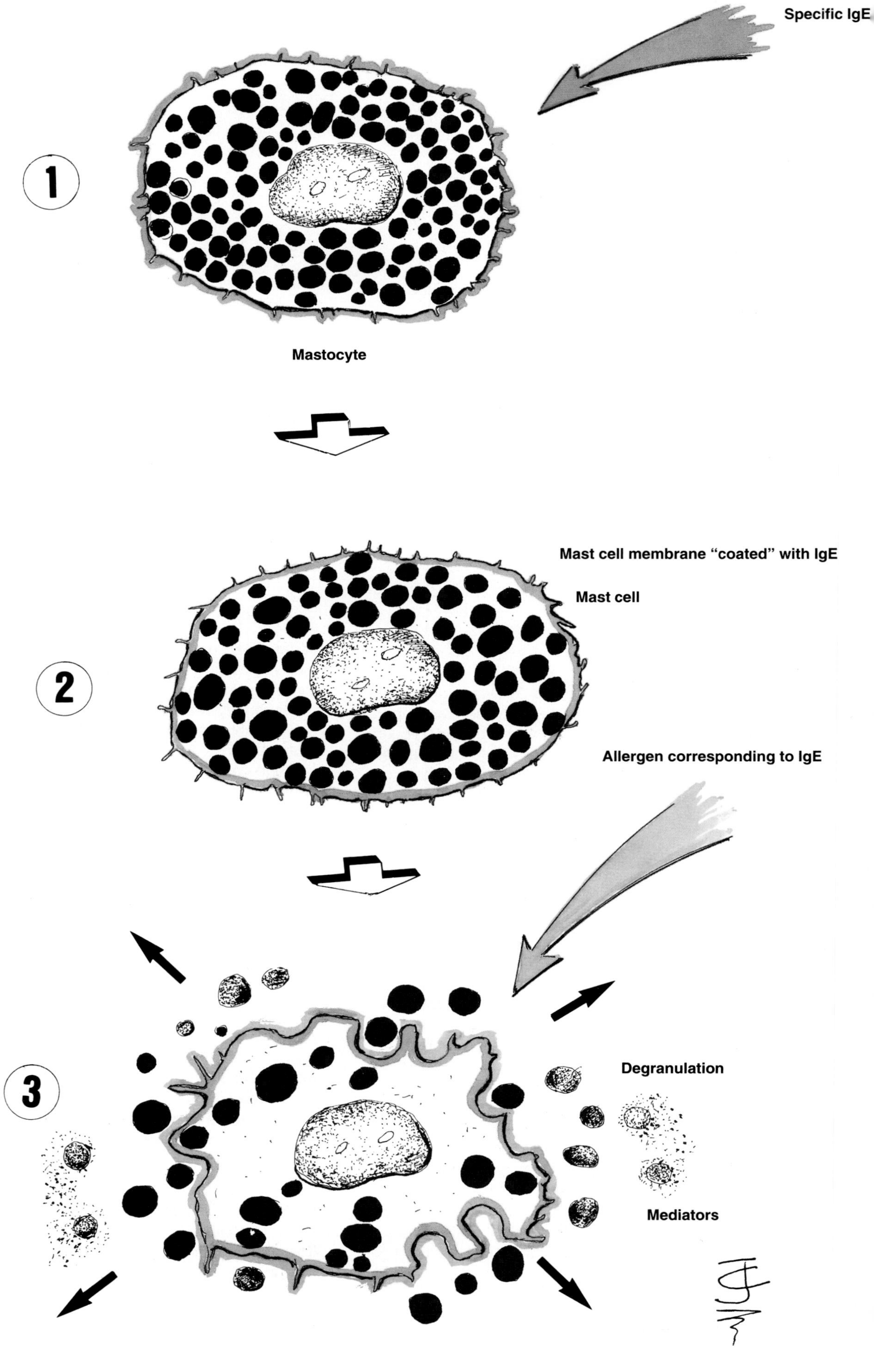

Specific IgE

1

Mastocyte

Mast cell membrane "coated" with IgE

Mast cell

2

Allergen corresponding to IgE

3

Degranulation

Mediators

Figure 42

1.12.2 Type I immediate allergic reaction or anaphylactic reaction (after Coombs and Gell)

This reaction, also called **anaphylactic**, comprises three elements **(Figure 42)**:
1. The **mast cells** in tissues, or the **basophils**, their equivalent in blood. These are the target cells.
2. The specific **IgE** immunoglobulin.
3. The **allergen** specific for an IgE.

Atopic or allergic individuals specifically synthesize more IgE antibodies for genetic reasons.

In ❶, mast cell or basophil containing many large granules. The arrow indicates contact with **specific IgE** (previously called **reaginic antibody**). In ❷, IgE is fixed to the mast cell membrane by a high affinity receptor (FcεRI). IgE is described as cytophilic or cytotropic because it fixes onto the target cell. If a patient is found to have 100 ng/ml of IgE in plasma, it is estimated that there are 4,000 molecules of IgE fixed per basophil. In ❸ is shown what happens when contact is made with allergen (green arrow). Mast cell or basophil granules leave the cell without destroying it: this is called **degranulation**. These granules contain highly potent **mediators**, especially histamine and heparin. In addition, a number of newly formed mediators, such as leukotriene C4 (LTC4), are also released.

Type I mechanism is responsible for the following diseases:
- Allergic asthma
- Seasonal (hay fever) or perennial allergic rhinitis
- Acute urticaria
- Anaphylactic shock (in particular after Hymenoptera stings, penicillin, and many other drugs). It should be taken notice that in case of drugs, type I mechanism is sometimes suspected but cannot always be confirmed.
- Certain digestive disorders such as angioneurotic edema (massive swelling of the face), urticaria, vomiting, etc. which are suspected to be of type I allergy.

Besides the mechanisms implying IgE antibodies, numerous non-specific factors are capable of triggering massive **release of histamine** by degranulation of mast cells, e.g., in allergy to cold, solar urticaria, heat urticaria, dermographism, reactions to some drugs (e. g., opiates, aspirin). When there is release of the same mediators by mast cells or basophils without involvement of specific IgE antibodies, the term of pseudo-allergic reaction is frequently used. Degranulation may also be triggered in non-specific manner by **histamine releasing factors** produced by other activated cells, such as T lymphocytes of monocytes **(Figure 48)**.

MAST CELL MEDIATORS

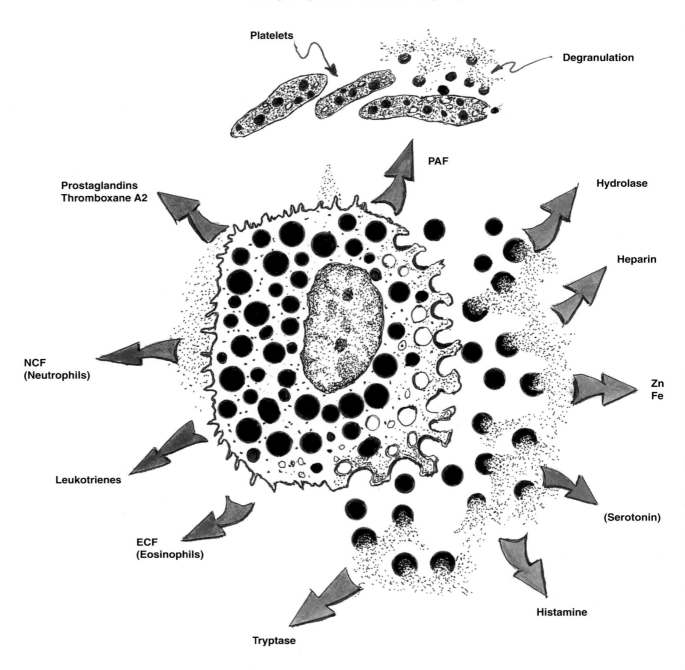

Platelets

Degranulation

PAF

Hydrolase

Prostaglandins
Thromboxane A2

Heparin

NCF
(Neutrophils)

Zn
Fe

Leukotrienes

(Serotonin)

ECF
(Eosinophils)

Histamine

Tryptase

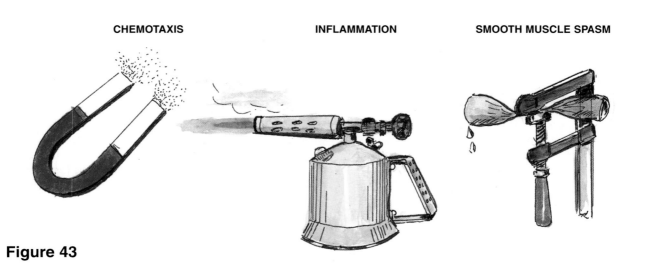

CHEMOTAXIS

INFLAMMATION

SMOOTH MUSCLE SPASM

Figure 43

1.12.2.1 Immediate hypersensitivity mediators (type I)

During an immune reaction, mast cells and basophils release mediators which have three kinds of effects: inflammation, bronchospasm and chemotaxis.

To be distinguished **(Figure 43):**

A. **Mediators contained in the granules** and released at time of degranulation (blue arrows, **Figure 43):**
- **Histamine:** increases vascular permeability, provokes spasm of smooth muscles, has a chemotactic effect on eosinophils, stimulates prostaglandin synthesis, stimulates the parasympathetic nerves, and mucus secretion . Its action is brief. It is inhibited by type H1 and, to a lesser extent, by type H2 antihistamines.
- **Serotonin:** causes contraction of smooth muscles and increases vascular permeability. Its role is lesser in man than in certain animal species.
- **Heparin:** an anticoagulant.
- **Various enzymes:** such as hydrolase and tryptase which activate C3 (activity blocked by heparin).

B. On the other hand, some **mediators, appear rapidly at the same time as degranulation** but are not linked to granules (red arrows, **Figure 43).**
- **Prostaglandins** among which PGF2 α and PG D2 contract bronchial smooth muscles while PG E2 dilates them.
- **Leukotrienes** C4, D4 and E4 make up the former **SRS-A (Slow Reacting Substance of Anaphylaxis).** They contract intensely bronchial smooth muscles, increase vascular permeability and facilitate migration of inflammatory cells.

Prostaglandins, thromboxanes, and leukotrienes are all inflammatory mediators produced by transformation of arachidonic acid. They are known collectively as **eicosanoids.**
- **Platelet-activating factor** (PAF) induces degranulation of platelets, which, in turn, release a number of mediators aggravating allergic reactions, in particular a mediator strongly chemotactic for eosinophils. PAF may also stimulate directly some inflammatory cells (e. g., basophils and eosinophils).
- A number of **chemotactic factors** is also observed, such as LTB4, ECF and NCF. **ECF** is a chemotactic factor for eosinophils, to be found among others in anaphylactic reactions. **NCF** is a factor chemotactic for neutrophils.

Biochemistry of these mediators is extremely complex, the more as the one or the other has the effect of increasing or impairing biological reactions. Chemotactic factors induce migration of cells such as neutrophils, eosinophils, and macrophages towards the sites of antigen-antibody reactions.

In turn, the migrating cells, also carrying receptors for immunoglobulins, may become stimulated and release a variety of mediators capable of encouraging the development of an inflammatory reaction and the appearance of tissue lesions. This is particularly observed during the late phase of type I reactions **(Figure 48).**

C. **Stimulated basophils and mast cells** are likewise able to **produce various cytokines** after some hours, such as IL-4, IL-5 and IL-3. In this way, they contribute to maintaining chronic allergic inflammation (see 1.12.5).

TYPE II ALLERGY

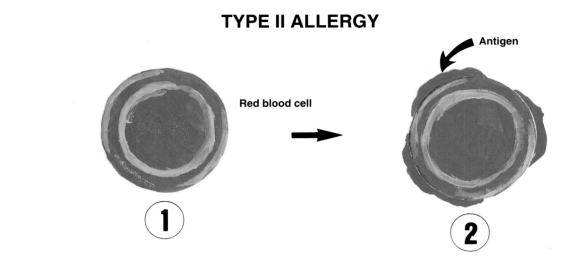

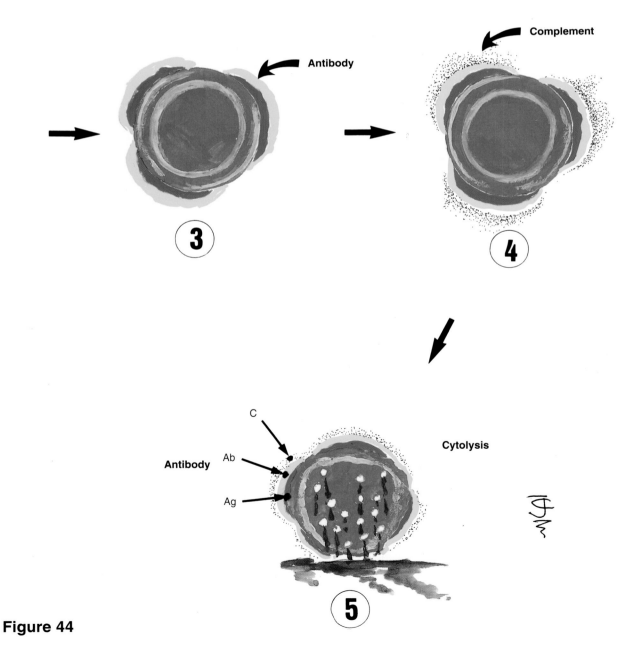

Figure 44

1.12.3 Type II immune reaction or cytotoxic reaction

In this type of reaction **(Figure 44)**, antigen adheres to a cell membrane, as e. g., the membrane of a red blood cell. The antigen may be a hapten, e.g., some drug such as cephalosporin, penicillin, etc.

In contrast to type I, antibody rather than antigen triggers the reaction, fixing onto the antigen which is itself fixed to the target cell. The responsible antibody is of the IgG or IgM class.

Figure 44 shows a red blood cell in ❶; in ❷ an antigen is fixed to its membrane. In ❸, an antibody becomes fixed to the antigen, which is itself fixed to the cell membrane. In ❹, complement is about to fix to this antigen-antibody complex and will trigger a violent cytolytic reaction. ❺ shows cytolysis with perforation of the cell membrane. These perforations are clearly visible under the electron microscope.

When complement is not involved in aggravating the reaction, there may simply be release of lysosomal enzymes from the target cells or opsonisation by a macrophage.

Numerous immunological reactions belong to type II, such as:
− Hemolytic disease of the newborn.
− Blood transfusion reactions by blood group incompatibility.
− Glomerulonephritis by auto-antibodies.
− Some types of hemolytic anemia, particularly drug-induced.
− Purpura by drug hypersensitivity.
− Masugi nephrotoxic nephritis.
− Drug-induced agranulocytosis.

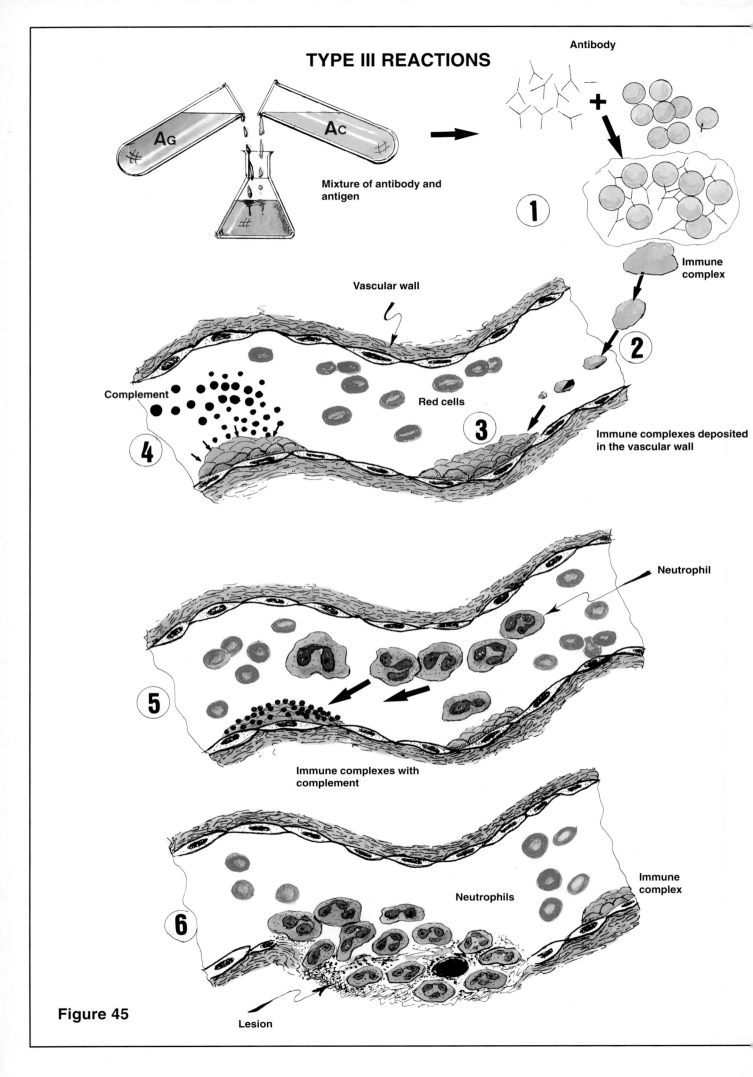

TYPE III REACTIONS

Antibody

A_G A_C

Mixture of antibody and antigen

1

Immune complex

2

Vascular wall

Complement

Red cells

3

Immune complexes deposited in the vascular wall

4

Neutrophil

5

Immune complexes with complement

6

Neutrophils

Immune complex

Lesion

Figure 45

1.12.4 Type III immune reaction or immune complex reaction

Reactions of type III involve formation of precipitating circulating antigen/antibody complexes in the blood, called **immune complexes or IC. Figure 45** shows the evolution of this mechanism.

In ❶, antigens and antibodies form immune complexes (IC) containing several antigens or several antibodies. The antibodies are bivalent and of IgG class, enabling them to "hook onto" several antigen molecules at once. Complexes ❷ mainly deposit in vascular walls ❸ or infiltrating glomerular membranes of the kidneys. Once fixed, they attract complement ❹. Complement attracts neutrophils ❺, in particular due to release of anaphylatoxins, which are powerful inflammatory mediators. The anaphylatoxins produced by complement activation induce degranulation of mast cells and basophils which, in turn, release many other highly active mediators. Vascular lesions with hemorrhages, thromboses, etc. appear at the site of the precipitation of immune complexes ❻.

When the type III reaction remains localized, a lesion known as **"Arthus phenomenon"** is observed.

ARTHUS PHENOMENON

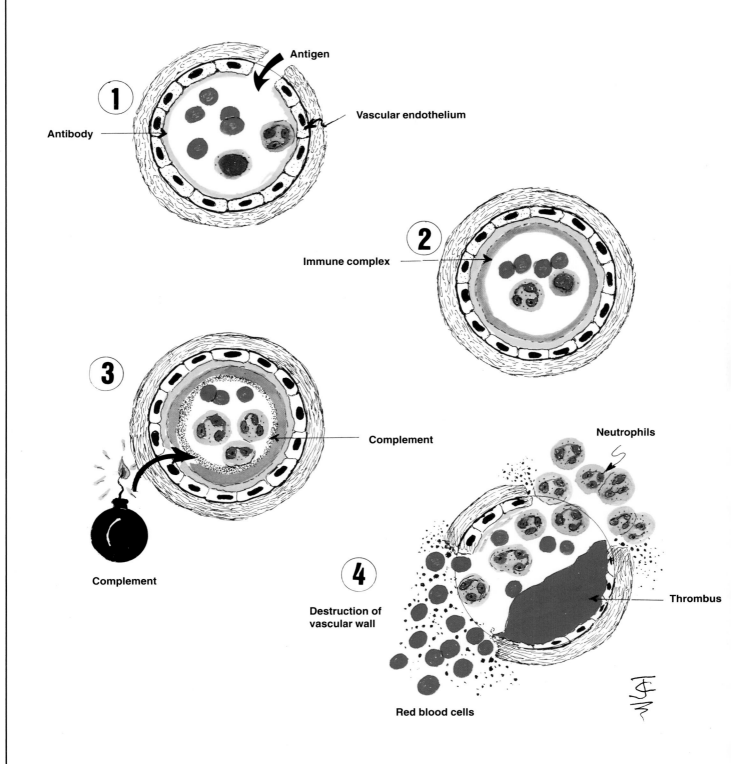

Figure 46

1.12.4.1 Arthus phenomenon

This is a type III allergic reaction. It is localized at the site of intradermal injection of an antigen in an individual carrying precipitating antibodies specific for this antigen. The Arthus phenomenon is illustrated in **Figure 46**. In ❶, the antibody is lining the vessel wall. An antigen, arriving locally in the vessel binds to the antibody, thus forming an immune complex. The immune complex (IC) deposits in the vessel wall ❷. Complement, required for the Arthus reaction to occur, fixes to this complex ❸ and acts like a "bomb" ignited by the immune complex.

A chemotactic factor attracting polymorphonuclears and various other inflammatory mediators are then released. In ❹, a vascularitis occurs with influx of polymorphonuclears which are releasing lysosomal enzymes. This causes localized destruction of the vessel wall with hemorrhage, diapedesis of polymorphonuclears, thrombosis, deposition of fibrin, localized edema, etc.

The main **diseases** caused by type III reactions include:
- Serum sickness.
- Collagen diseases, including lupus erythematosus.
- Glomerulonephritis, caused by immune complexes, as in malaria.
- Inflammation accompanying streptococcal infection.
- Allergic vascularitis.
- Some types of urticaria.
- Erythema nodosum.
- Blood disorders with hemolysis or thrombocytopenia.
- Rheumatoid arthritis, etc.

When the phenomenon is localized, and of the Arthus type, it leads to diseases such as **allergic aspergillosis, bird-fancier's lung, farmer's lung**, fever due to bacteria developing in **humidifiers**, etc. Drugs such as penicillins, phenacetin, and rifampicin may also provoke type III allergies.

TYPE IV REACTION

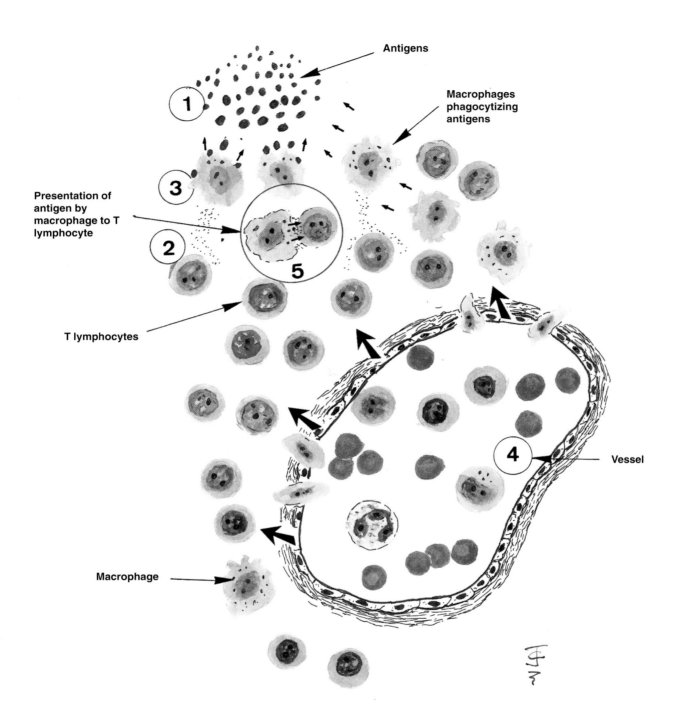

Antigens

Macrophages phagocytizing antigens

Presentation of antigen by macrophage to T lymphocyte

T lymphocytes

Macrophage

Vessel

Figure 47

1.12.5 Type IV immune reaction or delayed-type reaction.

In this type of reaction, the cause is not a circulating antibody. The allergic reaction is instead due to a **mechanism triggered by lymphocytes**. It is also known as **"cell-mediated hypersensitivity"** or **"delayed type hypersensitivity"** because the reaction appears late, within 24 to 48 hours after contact with antigen. The best-known example of this effect is the **tuberculin reaction**. After local injection of tuberculin in the skin of a sensitized individual, a reaction will appear 24 to 48 hours later.

Figure 47 shows a type IV allergic phenomenon: In ❶, antigens react with macrophages (in the skin with Langerhans cells) which present them to the one or the other specifically sensitized T lymphocyte ❺. This reaction produces a first wave of chemotactic mediators, which immediately attract non-specific lymphocytes ❷ and macrophages ❸. The latter appear on the "battle-field," coming from the vessels ❹ of the affected area. Under the microscope, the vessel is seen to be surrounded by a "sleeve" of lymphocytes and macrophages. Massive phagocytosis occurs where antigens and cells meet. Nonspecific T lymphocytes attracted secondarily to the site then release mediators, which direct the action of macrophages. Macrophages are also attracted to the site, where they are immobilized through the intervention of MIF. T lymphocytes stimulate phagocytosis and toxicity of the macrophages, which in turn release mediators (some interleukins) acting on proliferation of lymphocytes, and on their production of **lymphokines**.

Among lymphokines, the best-known include: migration inhibition factor **(MIF)**, which inhibits migration of macrophages and may be produced in vitro.

There is also a chemotactic factor for macrophages, a factor inducing phagocytosis, and a cytotoxic factor, capable of direct destruction of target cells without the intervention of complement.

Like the reaction observed in the late phase of type I reactions initiated by IgE and mast cells, the delayed reaction of type IV is due to a cascade of interactions which involve various cell types and different cytokines. However, in reactions of type IV, the cells participating in cellular infiltration are essentially mononuclear, i.e lymphocytes of type Th1, Ts (CD8) and monocytes. The involved lymphokines are likewise of type Th1, i.e., IL-2 and IFN γ. The kinetics are also different, as this type of reaction reaches its peak after 24–72 hours instead of 6–10 hours. A secondary basophil infiltration is observed occasionally, especially in skin reactions of type IV.

Effects of type IV reactions include:
- Contact dermatitis
- Defense against viruses, some bacteria, moulds, and parasites
- Rejection of grafts
- Autoimmune diseases
- Some drug allergies

The type IV mechanism probably plays a major role in the surveillance and elimination of neoplastic cells.

PATHOGENESIS OF IMMEDIATE AND LATE PHASE
IgE-DEPENDENT REACTIONS

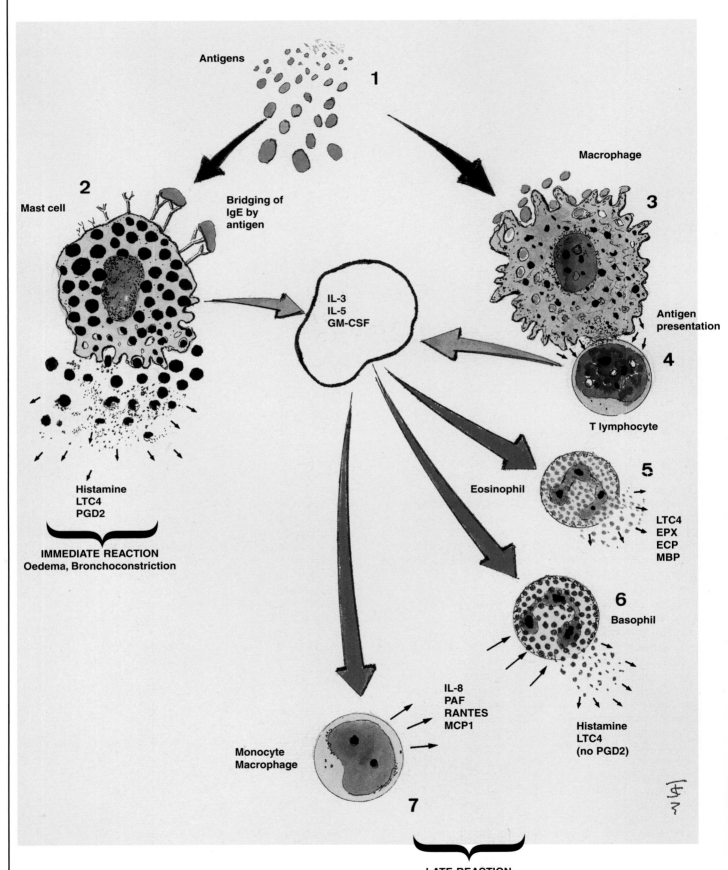

Figure 48

1.12.6 Allergic inflammation: A complex reality

The description of the four types of immune reactions according to Gell and Coombs corresponds well to the initial mechanisms triggering the various types of reactions but does not do justice to the physiopathological complexities which follow.

For example, type I reactions, called anaphylactic, are triggered by bridging specific IgE molecules bound to mast cell membranes, whereby the allergen performs the bridging **(Figure 48)**. The ensuing **immediate reaction** is characterized by the release of preformed mediators (e. g., histamine) or newly formed mediators (e. g., sulfidoleucotrienes: LTC4, LTD4, LTE4). This, however, is only part of the reaction.

This immediate phase, triggered by allergen in a few minutes, is often followed by a **late phase**, 6 to 8 hours later, without renewed allergen administration **(Figure 48)**. During the immediate phase of an IgE-dependent reaction, the originally involved cell is usually a tissue mast cell. It will quickly release or produce pharmacological mediators responsible for tissue edema through augmentation of vascular permeability and constriction of smooth muscles. Activated mast cells likewise produce chemotactic mediators which attract blood cells, particularly eosinophils and basophils, to the site of the reaction. After some hours the activated mast cells produce various cytokines, above all IL-3, IL-5 and GM-CSF, which produce pro-inflammatory activity.

A rather similar range of cytokines is, likewise, produced by Th2 cells, which are simultaneously activated by the allergen. Indeed, there will be no IgE specific for an allergen without concomitant clonal proliferation of allergen-specific T lymphocytes during the sensitization period. This cytokine production, called "Th2-like," has two effects: on the one hand it enhances the reactivity of basophils and eosinophils which are infiltrating the primary reaction site (**"priming phenomenon"**). On the other hand, it activates monocytes and tissue macrophages, which in turn produce additional mediators such as IL-8, RANTES, MCP-1 or PAF, which are all capable of triggering the release of histamine and other mediators by activated basophils. These factors have been globally described as **"histamine releasing factors."** Often a parallel activation of complement and production of anaphylatoxins C3a and C5a may add to the factors releasing a second wave of inflammatory mediators.

The late phase, involving cellular infiltration and the release of numerous mediators, including those released by eosinophils (e. g., ECP: Eosinophil Cationic Protein; MBP: Major Basic Protein) often plays a more important pathological role than the immediate phase, particularly in asthma. As seen in **Figure 48**, this inflammatory reaction does not strictly depend on the presence of IgE. Nonspecific activation of mast cells (as may be the case under the effect of certain drugs in **pseudo-allergic reactions**) or an independent activation of Th2 lymphocytes may lead to the same essentially eosinophil and basophil infiltration, to a similar release of mediators, and indeed to very similar symptoms. Thus, there is an evident clinical and physiopathological relationship between manifestations such as classical allergic asthma (called "extrinsic" and related to IgE reacting against inhalation allergens), "intrinsic" or endogenous asthma (evidently not related to the presence of IgE), and various pseudo-allergies, such as aspirin-induced asthma.

VARIOUS TYPES OF CYTOKINE-DRIVEN INFLAMMATION

Stimulated
lymphocytes:

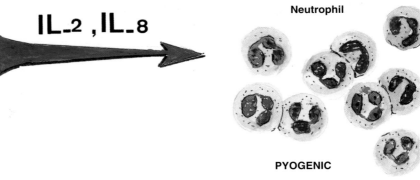

Neutrophil

IL_2 , IL_8

PYOGENIC

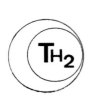

IL_3 , IL_5

Eosinophils

Basophils

ALLERGIC

IL_2 , IFNγ

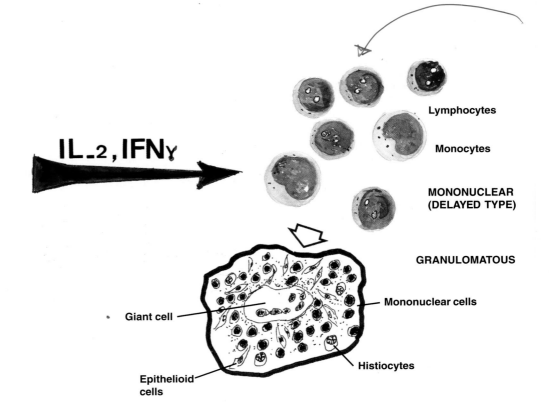

Lymphocytes

Monocytes

MONONUCLEAR
(DELAYED TYPE)

GRANULOMATOUS

Mononuclear cells

Giant cell

Histiocytes

Epithelioid
cells

Figure 49

It becomes more and more clear that the range of cytokines produced by T lymphocytes activated by allergens is directly responsible for the type of inflammatory reaction which follows. According to the participating cell types and to the resulting mediators, we presently distinguish between **(Figure 49)**:

a) **pyogenic** inflammation, involving neutrophils first and then leading to the formation of pus. In this type of inflammation, T lymphocytes leading the game seem to produce above all **IL-2** and **IL-8**.

b) **allergic** inflammation characterized by eosinophil and basophil infiltration, depending on Th2 lymphocytes producing above all **IL-3** and **IL-5**.

c) **lympho-monocytic** inflammation, depending on Th1 lymphocytes producing **IL-2** and interferon γ. In its chronic phase, this type of inflammation leads to **granulomatous** reactions, with differentiation of the mononuclear cells into histiocytes, epithelioid cells, giant cells, and activation of fibroblasts.

These distinctions between various patterns of inflammation and the related cytokines are oversimplified: the clinical reality is certainly more complex. Nevertheless, this conception helps us to better understand how the immunological defense reaction against the same external aggressor, e. g., lepra bacilli, may lead to very different clinical forms and evolutions of the disease. When the response involves mainly T lymphocytes of the Th1 type, the defense manifests itself in form of tissue granulomas **(tuberculoid leprosy)**. In contrast, when following a predominantly Th2 response, the disease evolves in largely disseminated form without localized tissue destruction **(lepromatous leprosy)**. Similarly, a Th1 response to Leishmania donovani is characterized by a localized granuloma and recovery from infection while a Th2 response leads to generalization (Kalaazar).

IMMUNOLOGICAL TOLERANCE

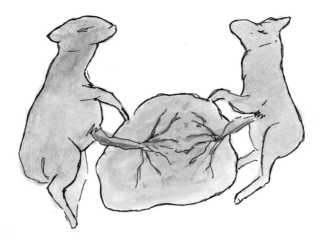

Heterozygotic twins sharing the same placenta and exchanging cells during embryonal development become tolerant of each other.

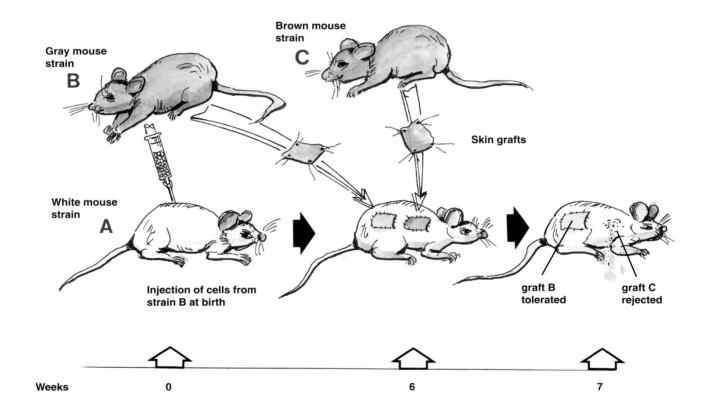

Gray mouse strain
B

Brown mouse strain
C

Skin grafts

White mouse strain
A

Injection of cells from strain B at birth

graft B tolerated

graft C rejected

Weeks   0   6   7

Figure 50

1.13 Immunological Tolerance

The immune system serves essentially as defense against foreign aggressors, such as bacteria or viruses but also against interior invaders (e. g., tumor cells). However, a mechanism is required which prevents the immune system from attacking the organism of which it is part, enabling it to recognize "self" from "non-self." Already in the beginning of the 20th century, Paul Ehrlich recognized the principle which permits the immune system to tolerate its own carrier. Ehrlich is the father of immunochemistry and coined the term "horror autotoxicus," the principle of which was later defined as **immunological tolerance**. In absence of this effect, the immune system may turn against its own organism, causing an **"auto-immune disease."**

Antigens native to the organism, i. e., antigens of the "self" are neither chemically nor structurally different from other antigens: they are, by the way, recognized by a different organism as "non-self" and rejected. Accordingly, **immunological tolerance of "self" is an acquired phenomenon, evolving during embryonal development** and maturation of the organism. This phenomenon is as specific as the immune response itself: it is only valid for the antigens which have induced it.

In a first observation of this natural phenomenon, it was seen that dizygotic sheep, with different genetic constitutions but sharing the same placenta during pregnancy, become tolerant of each other. This tolerance is maintained in adult life **(Figure 50 A).** The demonstration that tolerance may be induced experimentally by contact of an immature immune system with "nonself" has been brought about by Medawar in a spectacular way **(Figure 50 B).** When mice of strain A are inoculated at birth, at a moment where their immune system is still immature, with bone marrow cells of strain B, they become tolerant of all cells of strain B. When in adult age, skin grafts of strain B and of another strain C are performed, only grafts from strain C are rejected, as immunological tolerance against those has not been induced.

The experimental analysis of immunological tolerance phenomena has shown that several mechanisms, which are not mutually exclusive, may cause tolerance **(Figure 51–54).**

MECHANISMS OF IMMUNOLOGICAL TOLERANCE
I. CLONAL ELIMINATION

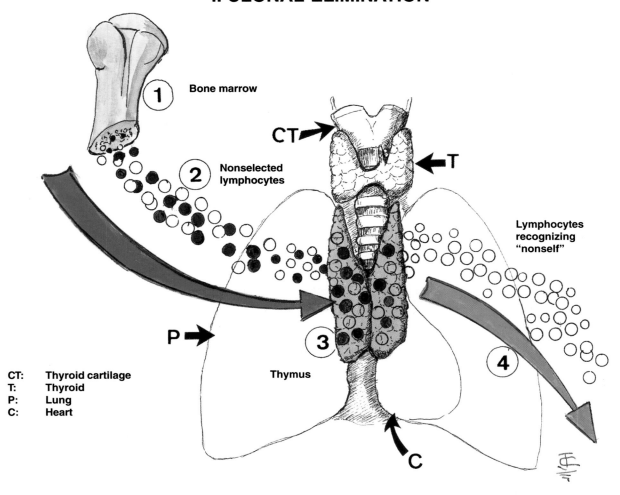

CT: Thyroid cartilage
T: Thyroid
P: Lung
C: Heart

Figure 51

Figure 51: T lymphocytes originating from bone marrow ❶ receive their education in the thymus ❷. The majority of them die rapidly there, in particular the ones able to recognize antigens of the "self" which are also present in thymus ❸. This is **"clonal elimination."** In contrast, alloreactive clones, e. g., those able to recognize the "non-self," survive and will colonize the various lymphoid organs ❹.

Figure 52: Tolerance, nevertheless, must be maintained during an entire life and must possibly also be acquired after environmental development. For this reason, an **immature lymphocyte** contacting the specific antigen which it recognizes might be stopped in its development and proliferation: this is the phenomenon of **clonal abortion.** By contrast, if antigen meets a fully mature lymphocyte, a normal immune response will follow with specific proliferation of the involved clone.

MECHANISMS OF IMMUNOLOGICAL TOLERANCE
II. CLONAL ABORTION

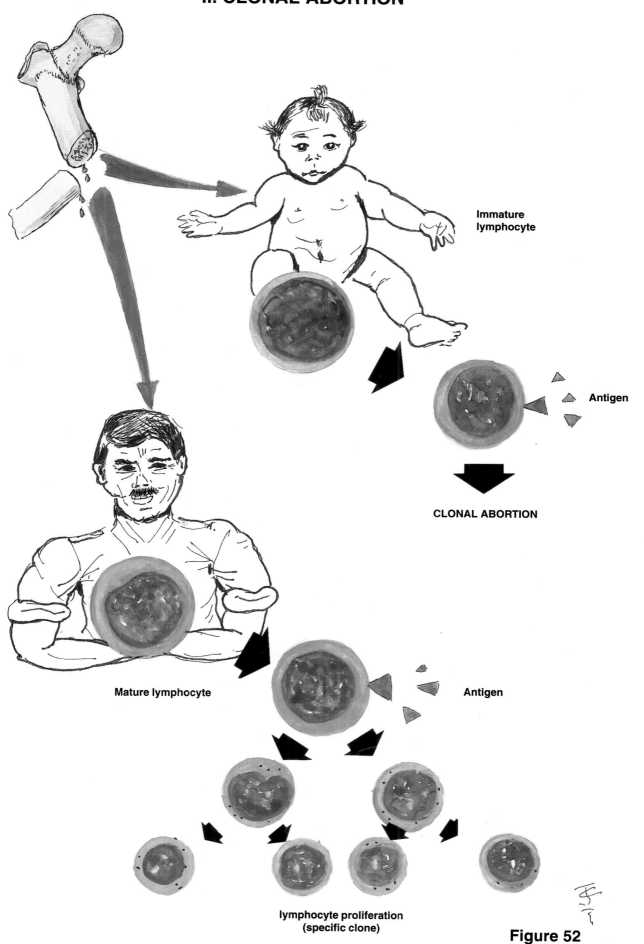

Immature lymphocyte

Antigen

CLONAL ABORTION

Mature lymphocyte

Antigen

lymphocyte proliferation
(specific clone)

Figure 52

MECHANISMS OF IMMUNOLOGICAL TOLERANCE
III. CLONAL ELIMINATION

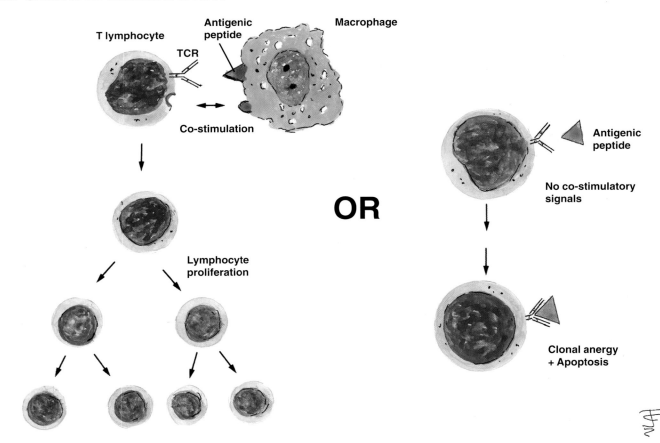

Figure 53

MECHANISMS OF IMMUNOLOGICAL TOLERANCE
IV. T CELL SUPPRESSION

Ly Th helper

Ag

Macrophage

Suppressor lymphokines (IL-10, TGF-β, etc.)

HALT

Suppressor T lymphocyte (Ts)

Figure 54

Figure 53: T lymphocytes require, in order to respond to stimulation and to be able to proliferate, that peptides originating from the antigen, recognized by T cell receptors (TCR), are presented by an accessory cell, which most of the time turns out to be a macrophage. **It is essential that the accessory cell send "co-stimulatory" signals.** If, on the other hand, the antigenic peptide is presented and recognized directly without co-stimulatory signals, the T lymphocyte will become unable to react. It has become **anergic.**

This phenomenon can be observed at an adult age, and even in an organism which has already shown an immune response against the antigen concerned. Identification of T cell epitopes, i.e., peptides recognized by the T lymphocytes, permits in principle their administration, inducing thereby induction of tolerance and specific desensitization. This procedure is presently being attempted in clinical trials for treatment of allergies and autoimmune diseases.

Figure 54: Certain lymphocytes activated by antigen produce cytokines preventing lymphocyte proliferation (e. g., IL-10, TGF-β). Such lymphocytes are naturally called **suppressors**. They largely explain the fact that immunological tolerance may be transmitted in some cases by cell injections from one tolerant animal to a non-tolerant animal.

T lymphocytes are made tolerant more easily than B lymphocytes: the majority of naturally acquired tolerance is based on that of T lymphocytes. In contrast, B lymphocytes are basically able to produce auto-antibodies against antigens of the "self" are often present even in the absence of a declared autoimmune disease. These are often a consequence of a breakdown in T lymphocyte tolerance against "self" antigens.

A better understanding of immunological tolerance permits new approaches in our therapy of autoimmune diseases and allergies, and it could greatly help us prevent rejection of transplanted organs.

INHERITANCE OF ATOPY
(Clinical manifestation: hay fever, asthma, atopic eczema)

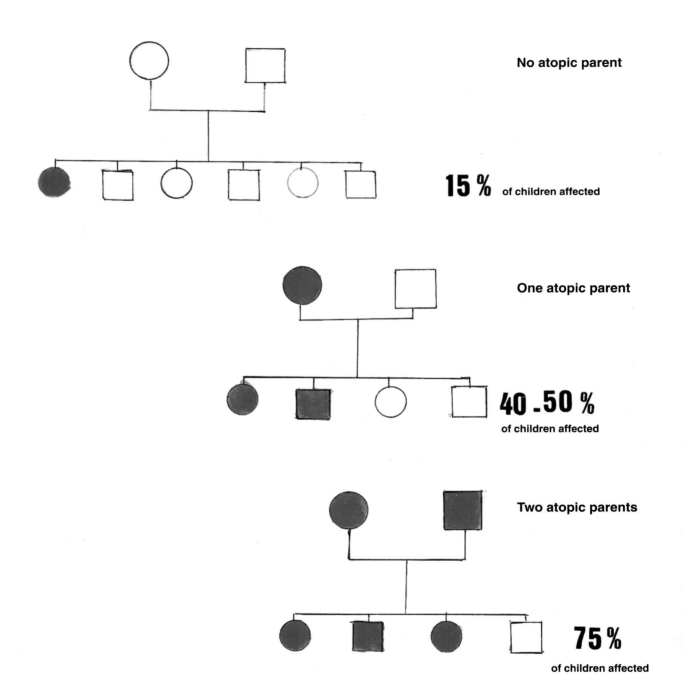

No atopic parent

15 % of children affected

One atopic parent

40 - 50 % of children affected

Two atopic parents

75 % of children affected

Figure 55

Part 2

Common Allergic Diseases

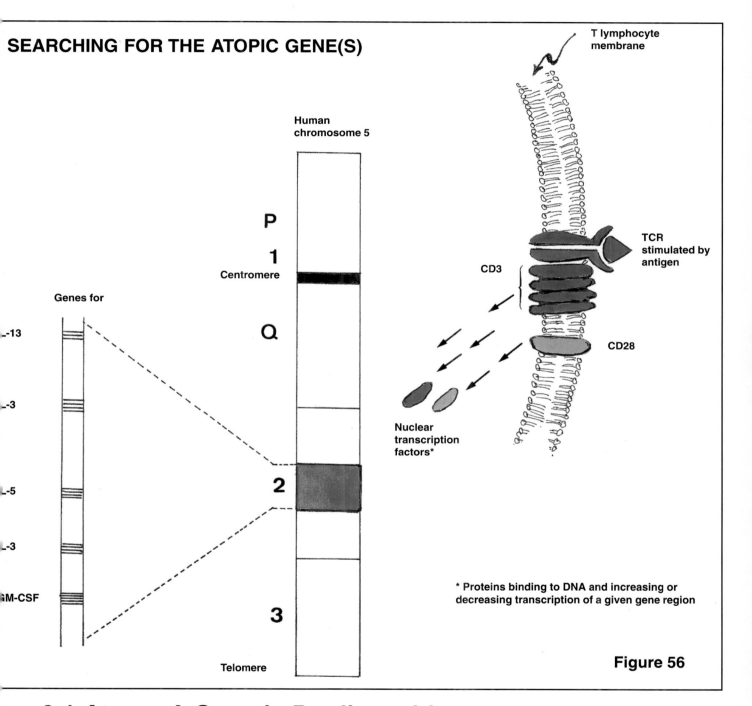

SEARCHING FOR THE ATOPIC GENE(S)

Human chromosome 5

P
1
Centromere

Q

2

3

Telomere

Genes for

L-13

L-3

L-5

L-3

GM-CSF

T lymphocyte membrane

TCR stimulated by antigen

CD3

CD28

Nuclear transcription factors*

* Proteins binding to DNA and increasing or decreasing transcription of a given gene region

Figure 56

2.1 Atopy: A Genetic Predisposition

Atopy (from the Greek ατωποσ: "not in its place") is a term coined by Cooke in 1923 to define the particular propensity of some individuals to develop certain typical allergic diseases, such as hay fever, asthma or atopic dermatitis. It has been proven that these diseases are more frequently encountered in some families, and consequently are under genetic influence.

Nevertheless, family tree analysis **(Figure 55)** with allergic trait transmission or studies performed in monozygotic twins do not show a homogeneous picture, which would be compatible with the inheritance of one single dominant or recessive gene. Atopy is more frequently present in children when both parents are atopic, but the disease may also jump one generation, when clinical manifestation of the disease is taken as criterion. In fact, what seems to be genetically inherited is not a clinical expression of allergic disease such as asthma or hay fever, but rather the capacity to develop such a disease, provided the individual concerned is exposed to certain allergens **early in life**. The definition of atopy has varied with time and with authors, which rendered the more difficult genetic analyses and their interpretation. Nowadays, **atopy is increasingly associated with a capacity to produce abnormal amounts of specific IgE following contact with minute amounts of allergens by inhalation or ingestion.**

Intensive research on the atopic gene(s) is currently under way. An English team recently described a system of autosomal dominant genes localized in region q13 of human chromosome 11, taking as readout criterion to define atopic individuals not the classical appearance of clinical diseases, but the presence of specific IgE against some of the common allergens. These results are, however, still controversial. Currently, the attention of researchers is increasingly focused on chromosome 5, which carries several genes responsible for expression of cytokines IL-4, IL-3, IL-5, IL-13 and GM-CSF **(Figure 56)**. These cytokines are typical "pro-allergic" factors, equally capable of fostering IgE production and enhancing mediator production in allergic inflammation. These cytokines, primarily produced by Th2 lymphocytes, are produced in large amounts in atopic patients, Therefore, it is plausible that genetic regulation apparent in atopic diseases is indeed related to the regulation of the expression of the "IL-4 family" of cytokines. At the molecular level, this regulation operates by a series of nuclear factors which either positively or negatively influence DNA transcription **(Figure 56)**.

Further genetic studies in well defined human populations, characterized by a high level of consanguine intermarriages, for example in the Pennsylvania Amish community, seem to confirm the association of genes located in the IL-4 area of chromosome 5 and hereditary atopy.

A precise identification of genes associated with atopy would certainly bear important practical consequences. On one hand, such a capability would permit early recognition of children "at risk" and the establishment of effective preventive measures. On the other hand, we can expect that knowledge of mechanisms regulating gene expression associated with atopy would permit discovery of specific therapeutic agents, preventing expression of the one or the other cytokine, as is already the case for some immunosuppressive and anti-inflammatory substances, like cyclosporin or FK 506.

2.2 Periodical or Seasonal Rhinitis: Hay Fever

Hay fever is an accepted term but it is, however, inappropriate, as it does not involve fever, and it is of course not hay but pollen that provokes the reaction.

The term **pollinosis** is more accurate. This precision is necessary, since the layman may easily confound hay fever with rhinitis caused by dust in barns and haylofts.

Classic hay fever is provoked by **grass pollens** (graminaceae). The most common of these are orchard grass, brome grass, velvet grass, meadow fescue, smooth stalked meadow grass, ray grass, wild oats, vernal grass, meadow foxtail, and timothy grass.

In *Western Europe,* graminaceae pollinate from May through the end of July, with a peak in June. Before this period, pollinosis may be caused by pollen from **trees**, especially birch (January to June). After grass pollination, pollens of **Compositae** may cause pollinoses (August and September). Artemisia, aster, chrysanthemum, golden rod, and ambrosia (also known as ragweed, the main culprit of pollinosis in the USA) are Compositae. Pollination varies from one region to another, and many plants play a more or less important part in pollinosis. A few additional examples are willow, alder, and hazel trees. Additional culprits include: pellitory, mimosa, and olive trees in southern Europe; nettle, plantain, clover, and cereals. In tropical countries, rice, tea, bamboo, and sugar cane also cause pollinosis.

The symptoms of hay fever include: itching of the eyes, nose, and the back of the throat, often very intense conjunctivitis, rhinitis with bouts of sneezing, obstruction, watery rhinorrhea and sometimes cough. Pollinoses are sometimes complicated by anosmia, inflammatory sinusitis and even asthma, which occurs more often in young patients. In addition to an early symptomatic phase there is in certain cases a late phase, occurring 6–10 hours after allergen contact, due to a local influx of eosinophils. Rhinoscopy, carried out during an acute episode, shows a characteristic picture: edematous and pale or lilac-colored mucosa, covered by clear secretions.

Very hot and dry weather provides the best conditions for the dispersion of pollens in the atmosphere and the consequent promotion of hay fever. In contrast, rain, of course, keeps pollens on the ground. Allergenic pollens are very small, invisible to the naked eye. They are called **anemophiles**, i.e., transported by wind. In contrast, the **entomophile** pollens, are more bulky and are carried by insects.

It is well known that hay fever sufferers have increased levels of eosinophils in their blood and in nasal secretions and, frequently, high IgE levels as well.

The most harmful activity for someone allergic to grass pollens is to mow grass during the period of pollination. Hay fever is the most characteristic allergic disease of type I.

Hay fever responds well to specific hyposensitization, supplemented, if necessary, by local (eye, nose) application of disodium cromoglycate or beclomethasone, and by the oral administration of antihistamines. Systemic administration of steroids is, in principle, not indicated in hay fever, except under exceptional circumstances (very severe hay fever, a pending marriage ceremony, university examinations, etc.)

2.3 Perennial or Non-Seasonal Rhinitis

Symptoms of non-seasonal allergic rhinitis resemble those of hay fever, but they do not follow a seasonal rhythm and are often less acute. Patients complain of frequent episodes of nasal obstruction, watery rhinorrhea, and bouts of sneezing. Headaches and hyperplasia or infection of the mucous membrane of the sinuses may complicate the picture.

When rhinitis is accompanied by asthma, it is easily neglected by the patient. In chronic infections, the picture is less typical. Nasal obstruction is the predominant symptom, sneezing is rare, rhinorrhea is less abundant and more often mucopurulent than watery; coughing is not uncommon, indicating tracheobronchial involvement.

Rhinoscopy shows varying images according to the histological lesions. The mucosa may be pale and edematous, or hypertrophic and congestive with mucopurulent secretions, or may even be atrophic.

Non-seasonal allergic rhinitis is most frequently caused by allergy to house dust mites, and is predominant in autumn. Other allergens may be responsible, such as animal fur (cats, dogs), horse or cattle hair, flour in bakeries, atmospheric moulds, drugs (in particular penicillin), various chemical substances (occupational allergies), and, perhaps, certain foods.

If allergy has an essential etiological role in non-seasonal rhinitis, other factors may play a role, such as infection or the mechanical blockade of sinuses.

2.3.1 Nasal polyposis

Nasal polyposis may be seen as a complication of non-seasonal rhinitis, but it is often the first sign of rhinitis. It generally consists of nasosinusal symptoms, with polyps originating in the maxillary or ethmoidal sinuses and extending to the nasal fossae at the end of a fine pedicle.

The origin and pathogenesis of such polyps are not yet elucidated. There is a syndrome known as Widal's triad, which comprises polyps, asthma, and aspirin intolerance, but its connection here is unclear. In addition, the importance of the allergic factor in polyposis is highly controversial.

Polyps are pale or pink, insensitive to palpation, have a softish consistency ("fish bladder" aspect) and must not be confounded with **adenoids**, which are fleshy exuberances of a lymphoid nature. When there might be confusion, it is important to ask the opinion of an ENT specialist.

Sometimes, it may be difficult to distinguish between lingering allergic rhinitis and chronic non-allergic rhinitis. Allergy should be suspected in particular in children. Treatment is the same for both non-seasonal allergic rhinitis and for hay fever: hyposensitization (less successful than in pollinosis), antihistamines, local corticosteroids (beclomethasone), and disodium cromoglycate. Antibiotics are justified for infectious episodes.

2.3.2 Removal of adenoids and tonsils

The question often asked, is whether or not to remove adenoids and tonsils. Bulky and irritating adenoids, responsible for continuous nasal obstruction, should be removed (adenoidectomy), if possible. In contrast, tonsillectomy should be reserved for chronic and/or complicated infections (otitis), after the failure of prolonged and correct medical treatment. Cases of asthma have been known to develop after inappropriate tonsillectomy.

2.4 Asthma

Actually, there is no definition of asthma which has been unanimously accepted by specialists. However, an international consensus recently defined asthma to be **a respiratory disease characterized by:**
1) **Bronchial obstruction which is not always entirely reversible**
2) **Inflammation of the airways**
3) **Bronchial hyperreactivity to various stimuli.**

Briefly, it may be stated that three key elements are involved to a variable extent and may be more or less reversible: spasm of bronchial muscles, mucosal edema, and mucus hypersecretion.

2.4.1 Asthma and bronchial hyperreactivity

With very few exceptions, symptomatic asthma affects only patients with non-specific or non-allergenic bronchial hyperreactivity (NABH), i.e., an exaggerated sensitivity of the bronchial wall.

This hypersensitivity is manifested in abnormal permeability of the mucosae towards antigens, ortho-parasympathetic imbalance (orthosympathetic being bronchodilator and parasympathetic being bronchoconstrictor), hypertrophy and hyperexcitability of the bronchial muscles.

If bronchial hyperreactivity is accompanied by sensitization to an allergen, with formation of specific antibodies (IgE), exposure to this allergen may trigger an asthma attack. **This is extrinsic, allergic, or atopic asthma. Atopy** may also be defined as a tendency to develop symptoms of immediate type I hypersensitivity, such as asthma, hay fever, urticaria, and eczema after contact with allergens.

In other forms of asthma, no symptoms or proof of allergy, such as specific IgE, may be found. Attacks occur after exposure to non-specific irritants (cigarette smoke, cold air, physical exercise, etc.), or even without any apparent cause. This is called **intrinsic asthma.**

ARACHIDONIC ACID DERIVATIVES

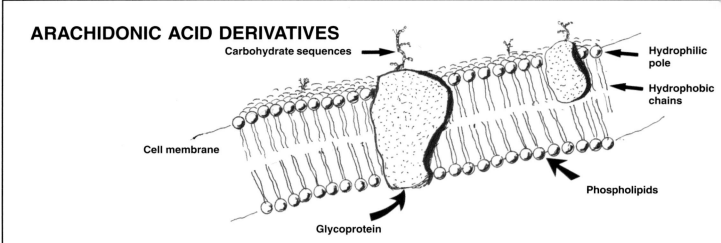

Carbohydrate sequences

Hydrophilic pole

Hydrophobic chains

Cell membrane

Phospholipids

Glycoprotein

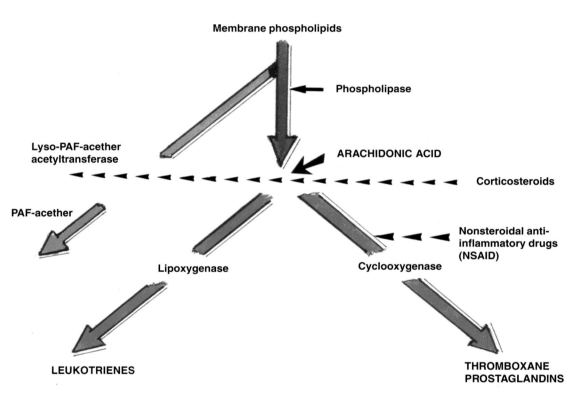

Membrane phospholipids

Phospholipase

Lyso-PAF-acether acetyltransferase

ARACHIDONIC ACID

Corticosteroids

PAF-acether

Nonsteroidal anti-inflammatory drugs (NSAID)

Lipoxygenase

Cyclooxygenase

LEUKOTRIENES

THROMBOXANE PROSTAGLANDINS

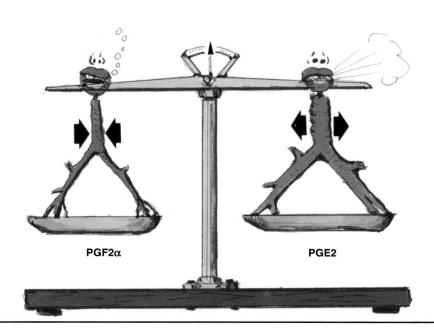

PGF2α

PGE2

Figure 57

Nevertheless, the level of total IgE is often increased, which could mean that so-called "intrinsic" asthma is simply extrinsic asthma for which the allergen remains unknown. Another possibility is that intrinsic asthma is triggered by the interaction of T cells with antigens (e.g., moulds or bacteria), triggering eosinophilia and the release of secondary mediators similar to the ones observed in the late phase of immediate reactions due to IgE. Whatever the case, non-specific and specific stimuli can both maintain bronchial hyperreactivity.

Some individuals are allergic, but are free of bronchial hyperreactivity; aggression by an allergen does not cause asthma in such individuals, but other allergic manifestations, such as rhinitis, urticaria, and conjunctivitis.

Bronchial tonus follows a circadian rhythm and is at its most fragile towards the end of the night, a time at which many asthmatics have problems. This factor is important in the treatment of asthma, because the drug prescribed must last long enough to cover this most unstable period. The autonomous nervous system also plays an important role in regulation of bronchial diameters, but the mechanism is not clearly understood. Two non-allergic conditions may trigger asthma, and should be kept in mind:
1. intolerance of certain drugs: **aspirin** in particular, and **beta-blockers**;
2. **gastroesophageal reflux:** rather frequent, manifested in pyrosis, particularly when lying down or leaning forwards. Further research seems necessary.

Sensitive nerve endings are found between bronchial cells, in the nose, larynx, and pharynx. The stimulus is directed towards the central nervous system, and travels from there to the peripheral target organ.

Destruction of the bronchial epithelium, frequent in chronic asthma, favors stimulation of the underlying nerves. Stimulation of parasympathetic nerves (vagus nerve) causes bronchial contraction, while excitation of sympathetic fibers leads to relaxation.

The cells of smooth muscles contain not only beta-adrenergic receptors, the stimulation of which by catecholamines causes bronchial relaxation, but also alpha receptors, stimulation of which causes bronchial contraction.

Various vagolytic drugs, such as ipratropium, are very effective in certain forms of asthma.

2.4.2 Mediator cascade and inflammation

During an IgE-dependent reaction, a whole series of mediators is released, not only by mast cells and basophils, but also by other cells. Mediators may be classified according to their origin: **membrane mediators** of lipid origin (PAF, leukotrienes, prostaglandins, thromboxane A2), and **granular mediators** such as eosinophil, cationic proteins, and above all histamine.

Mediators may also be grouped according to their principal function: **chemotaxis** (ECF, NCF, LTB4), **cytolysis** (MBP, EPO, eosinophil EDN/EPX), **vasoactivity** (prostaglandins, leukotrienes).

No classification can, however, account for the complexity of interactions between all these substances, since one and the same mediator can be secreted by different cells, act on different cells, and interact with other mediators.

The following description attempts to place the main elements of this field within a broader context wihtout implying a chronological or hierarchic order.

2.4.2.1 Preformed mediators
Histamine is stored mainly in basophil and mast cell granules. By fixing to H1 receptors, it induces bronchoconstriction, pulmonary vasoconstriction, increased capillary permeability, increased production of nasal mucus, and a chemotactic effect on neutrophils.

Chemotactic factors have been described for eosinophils **(ECF)** and for neutrophils **(NCF)**: the latter, of mast cell origin, also induce neutropenia.

Granules of eosinophils contain in particular **MBP** (Major Basic Protein), which is the central crystalloid of granules, **ECP** (Eosinophil Cationic Protein), **EDN/EPX** (eosinophil derived neurotoxin identical to eosinophil protein-X), and **EPO** (Eosinophil Peroxidase). All these substances are strongly cytotoxic.

2.4.2.2 Newly formed mediators
Prostaglandins and **thromboxane (Figure 57)** are derived from arachidonic acid by the cyclo-oxygenase pathway, which is blocked by aspirin, NSAIDs, and corticosteroids.

PGD2 has various local inflammatory properties, PGE2 is **bronchodilating** and **vasodilating**, while **PGF2** is **bronchoconstricting** (more powerful than histamine). In asthma, there appears to be an imbalance between PGE2 and PGF2. PGD2, a potent thrombolytic, is synthesized in large amounts by mast cells. **TXA2** is a potent vasoconstrictor and platelet aggregating agent. **Prostacyclin** (PGI2) is also synthesized by this route, in particular in endothelial cells: it is a powerful vasodilator and anti-aggregating agent for platelets by stimulation of the adenylate cyclase-cyclic AMP system.

Leukotrienes (LT) are synthesized from arachidonic acid by the lipoxygenase pathway, which may be blocked by corticosteroids. LTA4, a common precursor, is converted, depending on the cells involved, into **LTB4** and/or **LTC4** and its metabolites **LTD4** and **LTE4** (the last three form SRS-A or "slow-reacting substance of anaphylaxis").

LTs are **bronchoconstrictors** and LTC4, for example, is 100–1,000 times more powerful than histamine. In addition, LTB4 is a potent chemotactic agent for neutrophils, and it might regulate the activity of NK cells: LTC4 and LTD4 reduce mucociliary clearance and increase mucus production.

PAF (or PAF-acether) is produced by the action of phospholipase A2 on membrane phospholipids. It is one of the most powerful platelet-aggregating agents known, but also one of the most powerful chemotactic factors for eosinophils. Its bronchoconstricting action is exerted via cell and platelet mediators, the release of which it stimulates.

PGs and LTs are also involved in general inflammatory processes. In addition, **cytokines** produced by T lymphocytes and monocytes attracted to the site of inflammatory reactions or produced by stimulated mast cells **(Figure 48)** play an important role. Some of these cytokines "prime" inflammatory cells for increased production of mediators (e.g., IL-3, IL-5, GM-CSF), others may act direct-

ASTHMA
(for patient information)

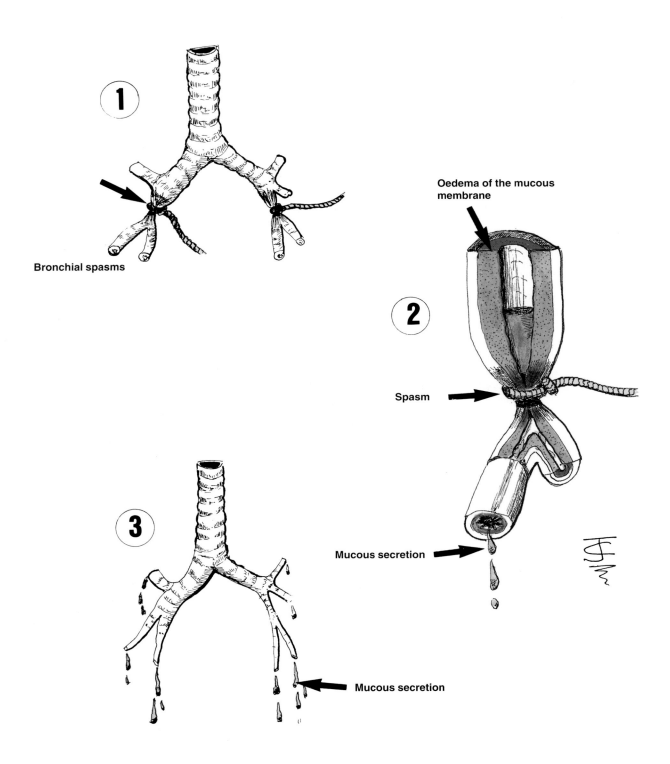

Figure 58

ly to stimulate the same cells (histamine releasing factors, e. g., IL-8, MCP-1, RANTES and so on).

In the first stage of inflammation, that is in the immediate phase of IgE-dependent allergic reactions, edema occurs as a result of the increased circulation and permeability of the microcirculation, due to the release of histamine and leukotrienes. PGD2, LTC4, and LTD4 are potent vasodilators, of long duration for PGs and short duration for LTs. Furthermore, PGE2 blocks release of noradrenaline from sympathetic nerve endings.

In the second stage of inflammation, e. g., in the late phase of IgE-dependent allergic reactions, the invasion of inflammatory cells is observed. These cells are attracted by numerous chemotactic mediators, including arachidonic acid derivatives, mainly LTB4. Additionally, LTB4 provokes exocytosis of lysosomes. In contrast, derivatives generated by cyclo-oxygenase do not have any chemotactic activity. On the contrary, they act rather by increasing cyclic AMP, which inhibits the release of lysozymes, histamine, LTs and lymphokines. PGE2 inhibits the metabolism of leukocytes, phagocytosis, cytotoxicity, and certain lymphocyte functions.

The main inflammatory cells attracted to the reaction site, be they eosinophils, T lymphocytes, monocytes, or in some cases basophils, produce in turn mediators, under the influence of various cytokines **(Figure 48).**

As seen, **asthma is therefore produced by a complex interaction of numerous cells and mediators**.

2.4.3 Bronchial obstruction. Histopathological stages of asthma

Three phases are distinguished in bronchial obstruction **(Figure 58)**, which are partly overlapping:
1) **Bronchospasm**
2) **Bronchial obstruction by inflammatory edema** of the bronchi, to which mucus secretion is added
3) **Subacute or even chronic inflammation.**

These phases are initially triggered by mediators released by mast cells, either during an IgE-allergen interaction or during the non-specific degranulation of mast cells (e. g., in exercise induced asthma, an infection, etc.).

Figure 58 emphasizes three elements of bronchial obstruction: spasm, edema, and thick secretion. These are the targets of symptomatic treatment. This is where the impact of symptomatic treatment lies and is **the pattern to be explained to the patient to gain his or her cooperation.**

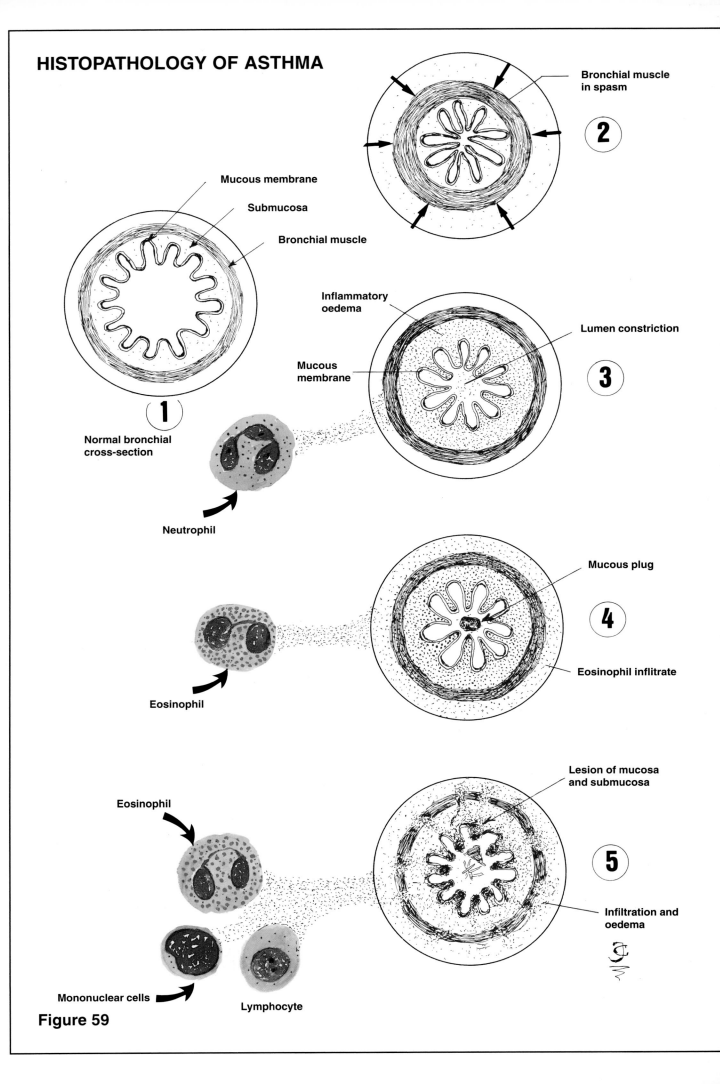

HISTOPATHOLOGY OF ASTHMA

Bronchial muscle in spasm

2

Mucous membrane

Submucosa

Bronchial muscle

Inflammatory oedema

Lumen constriction

Mucous membrane

3

1

Normal bronchial cross-section

Neutrophil

Mucous plug

4

Eosinophil inflitrate

Eosinophil

Lesion of mucosa and submucosa

Eosinophil

5

Infiltration and oedema

Mononuclear cells

Lymphocyte

Figure 59

Figure 59 shows the histopathological sequences of asthma, as defined upon experimental provocation.

❶ is a reference picture and shows a normal bronchial cross-section, with mucous membrane, submucosa, and bronchial muscle.

❷ Bronchospasm: This **first phase**, called the early phase, is short-lived and manifests by increased airway resistance. It occurs 10–15 min after spasmogenic contact with the triggering stimulus. At this stage, bronchial obstruction is reversible, either spontaneously or by sympathomimetic bronchodilators. This bronchospasm is attributed essentially to histamine released by degranulation of mast cells, and to LTC4 production. It may be prevented by disodium cromoglycate or to a lesser extent by an H1-antihistamine. At this point, mast cells additionally release a neutrophil chemotactic factor (NCF) and LTB4. This chemotactic action triggers the start of an inflammatory reaction.

The **second phase** of asthma, is, of course, called the **late phase**. Bronchospasm is aggravated by an inflammatory edema of mucosa and submucosa. The reaction appears 5–8 hours after spasmogenic contact. It may last several days, and is much more serious than the first phase.

The inflammatory reaction only regresses slowly. In ❸ is shown the invasion of neutrophils attracted by activation of mast cells. In ❹ is shown the appearance of eosinophils. Leukotrienes and prostaglandins play a major part in this late phase, causing bronchial spasm and the aggravation of edema of mucosa and submucosa. This reaction is sensitive to corticosteroids, which inhibit the metabolism of arachidonic acid and the production of cytokines. Plugs of mucus impregnated with polynuclear cells form during this phase.

A **subacute** or **chronic third phase** then follows, accompanied by **severe inflammation** and massive infiltration of eosinophils and mononuclear cells. Besides their cytotoxic mediators (MBP and others), which are responsible for cytolysis of cells in the bronchial epithelium **(Figure 6)**, eosinophils also release leukotrienes which maintain bronchoconstriction. Consequently, the beneficial effect of a treatment that checks or blocks the eosinophil invasion is self-evident. Steroids and some antihistamines such as cetirizine, seem to act at this level. These three phases may be separated experimentally. In clinical practice, however, asthma often appears as chronic bronchial inflammation accompanied by bronchospastic episodes.

2.5 Urticaria and Angioneurotic Edema

Acute urticaria lasting from a few hours to a few days, is distinguished from **chronic urticaria,** which may persist for weeks or even months, often with intermittent remission periods. The first form is often allergic, the second is rarely so.

Urticaria may appear in several forms, but it is always accompanied by papular lesions ("nettle wheals"). Papules may be small, medium-sized, or may appear in patches. Urticaria may erupt anywhere on the body, and is characterized by **violent pruritus**, often accompanied by lesions due to scratching.

A specific form of acute allergic and edematous skin reaction is **angioneurotic edema**, or **Quincke's edema**: facial swelling with edema of lips, eyelids (eyes in slits), and sometimes the back of throat and pharynx (in severe forms), but without pruritus. Angioneurotic edema may be familial and **genetically inherited**, due to a deficiency in C1-esterase inhibitor.

There are several forms of urticaria. In acute allergic urticaria and angioneurotic edema, a food or drug allergen, hymenoptera stings, pneumallergens such as pollens ("meadow dermatitis"), allergies to animal hair, etc. are sometimes detected as the cause . Excessive nervousness is often involved, if not as primary etiology, then at least as an additional triggering factor. Some forms of urticaria are of physical origin, such as **solar urticaria, cold urticaria,** and **delayed pressure urticaria**.

The cause of chronic urticaria is in general not allergic and results from complex immunological or neuroendocrinological disorders, such as the deregulation of complement, circulating immune complexes in neoplasms, autoimmune diseases, infections such as mononucleosis, and digestive disorders such as gastritis. There is also **photoallergic urticaria**, provoked by so-called photosensitizing drugs such as phenothiazines. These drugs are transformed in the skin under the influence of the sun's ultraviolet rays, and release histamine directly or indirectly.

The pathology and etiology of chronic urticaria pose very different problems which are poorly understood.

The best way to treat urticaria is undoubtedly to prevent exposure to the responsible allergen but as a practical matter in the majority of cases the allergen cannot be identified. Treatment is based essentially on antihistamines. Drowsiness caused by some antihistamines is sometimes advantageous, as in nocturnal pruritus, but this secondary effect, bothersome in daytime, is almost completely eliminated in the most recent generation of antihistamines such as terfenadine, cetirizine and levamizole. Corticosteroids are only prescribed under exceptional circumstances. An underlying disease accompanied by urticaria should be suspected and carefully investigated (e. g., infectious mononucleosis), as numerous medical problems may be accompanied by urticaria.

The use of γ-globulin treatment sometimes yields interesting results for still unknown reasons. It has been postulated that when urticaria is due to small immune complexes which have not been eliminated, therapeutic γ-globulins "bring them down," and permit them to be eliminated by macrophages. In some cases, chronic urticaria has been associated with the presence of anti-IgE or anti-IgE receptor antibodies.

2.6 Contact Dermatitis

Contact dermatitis is an eczema localized at the site of application of a non-tolerated substance called allergenic, (e. g., in nickel allergy due to metal buttons of jeans, earrings, watch straps, etc.). This is a type IV delayed type allergy. Identification of the allergen is often difficult, and requires detailed history taking. As is well known, allergologists and dermatologists perform epicutaneous tests known as **patch tests** for this purpose. These consists in applying on the skin the suspected substance for a period of 2–3 days with a special adhesive patch. Unfortunately, it is not always easy to interpret the results of these tests. Reactions caused by irritation or burning should not be mistaken for clear signs of allergy.

For this reason, carefully calculated concentrations in neutral diluents are used in these tests. Allergenic substances encountered include: drugs (e. g., chloramphenicol, penicillin or neomycin ointments, etc.), cosmetics (shampoos, dyes, nail polishes, deodorants, etc.), exotic woods, epoxy resin glues, foods (chicory, artichokes, etc.), metal jewelry, etc. Altogether a considerable number of substances. Allergens are most frequently **haptens**, which combine with skin proteins to form complete allergens. There are specialized publications containing long lists of allergenic substances as well as concentrations and diluents to be used in patch tests. Contact eczema poses sometimes difficult problems for treatment, as the only effective method is to avoid the allergen involved.

Hairdressers and those individuals involved in manufacturing dyes, paints, adhesives, synthetic resins, oleoresins, antibiotics, as well as masons (cement chrome), etc., are particularly affected. Some forms of contact eczema are recognized by law as occupational diseases.

Contact allergy is a field belonging to the dermatologist.

2.7 Atopic Dermatitis (or atopic eczema)

Individuals with an increased tendency to synthesize IgE in response to allergenic stimuli are called **atopic**. Atopic dermatitis is often the first allergic manifestation in small children, and predominates in the bends of elbows and knees and on the cheeks. A hereditary allergic background is often present. This form of eczema heals between the ages of 3 and 4 years, or at puberty in numerous cases. Atopic eczema often causes localized areas of thickened skin due to scratching; these become easily superinfected, as the itching can often be quite intense.

Asthma may frequently occur while eczematous skin lesions disappear: it is often heard that "eczema has gone, but now asthma has taken its place." It should be well explained to the parents that this is not the doctor's fault! In the light of our experience regarding atopic eczema, we always recommend that a dermatologist be consulted, as many skin lesions may sometimes simulate eczema. Biopsies may become necessary for diagnostic purposes.

In about 30% of cases, attacks of atopic eczema may be brought on in connection with food allergies (e.g., milk, egg). Allergy against house dust mites is often the responsible culprit. These possible causes of exacerbation have to be carefully looked for.

Scratching and superinfections should, of course, be prevented. The wearing of irritating clothing (polyesters) and the excessive use of local corticosteroids should be avoided. Useful advice may be obtained in this respect from dermatologists. Oral antihistamines are useful to alleviate pruritus.

Despite the development of numerous theories, the physiopathology of eczema is still remarkably little understood. Researchers are currently focusing on Langerhans cells, which are thought to be involved in eczema, because these cells possess abundant receptors for IgE. Once in contact with allergen distributed after ingestion or following direct skin contact, Langerhans cells present the allergen to T lymphocytes. They may also be directly stimulated to produce inflammatory cytokines, which are responsible for eczematous lesions. Atopic eczema is often accompanied by very high IgE levels. In babies, an elevated IgE level is taken as a reliable predictive sign for the development of asthma and/or hay fever in later life.

2.8 Farmer's Lung and Other Type III Immune Complex Diseases (extrinsic alveolitis)

Farmer's lung is a condition which has become rare, affecting farm laborers who handle mouldy hay. It originates from poor conditions of cereal storage, involving lots of dust and humidity. Farmer's lung occurs mainly in rainy regions and semi-mountainous areas such as Wales, or Cantal in France. It appears mainly in autumn and winter and affects above all adult males. The condition sets in gradually, and takes the form of a respiratory problem accompanied by fever and dyspnea, i.e., a condition resembling influenza, appearing 8–10 hours after handling mouldy hay and straw. The patient presents with fever, shivering, chest pains, lassitude, sweating, headaches, and coughing, sometimes accompanied by hemoptysis. Clinically, fine auscultatory chest creeps may be present. In typical forms, the chest X-ray shows miliary infiltrates and micronodules. Later, pulmonary fibrosis appears progressively when the disease reaches a chronic stage. There is also impairment in alveolar gas diffusion (so called restrictive syndrome) and, in the most advanced cases, an alveolar-capillary block, which leads to chronic pulmonary heart failure.

Microorganisms responsible for farmer's lung are moulds, above all Micropolyspora faeni, and Thermoactinomyces vulgaris. Specific **precipitins** are found in the blood, especially antibodies of the IgG class. This disease is classified as a type III allergy.

Bird-fancier's lung, which is fairly common, is another disease of the same type, found especially among pigeon breeders. According to the case, serum contains precipitins against the serum proteins of pigeon, parrot, chicken, pheasant, turkey, and related animals.

Allergic bronchopulmonary aspergillosis (ABPA), caused by Aspergillus fumigatus, is accompanied by pulmonary infiltrates and elevated IgE levels. It is, in fact, a combination of type I allergy with type III allergy. The following type III conditions are much less common: duck fever (duck feathers), cheesemaker's disease (moulds or Acarus siro), bagassosis (sugar cane moulds), suberosis (cork), sequoiosis (redwood sawdust), inhalation of pituitary powder (in diabetes insipidus), corn-handler's disease and, more recently discovered, the disease caused by humidifiers (contamination of the water container by bacteria or moulds).

All these diseases have in common the presence of specific serum **precipitins**. However, in some of these diseases, the presence of IgG precipitins does not alone suffice to explain the lesions, because such IgG antibodies are also encountered in apparently healthy individuals exposed to the same allergens (e. g., pigeon breeders). The association of a type IV allergy is then postulated to explain the pathology.

SKIN TESTS IN ALLERGY

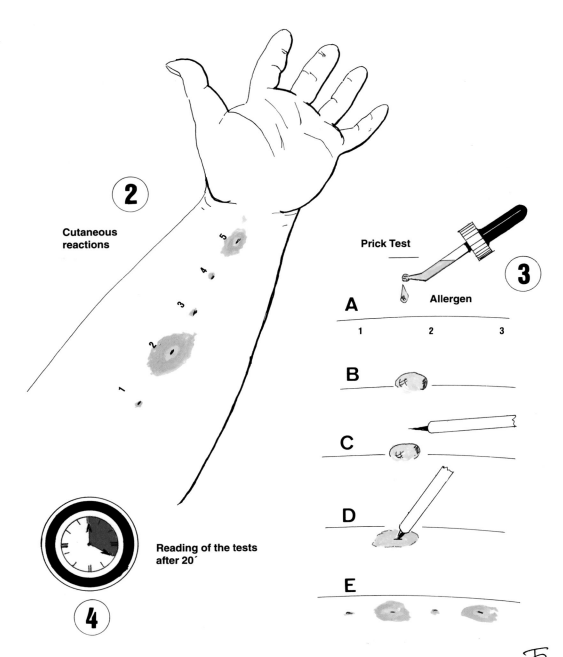

1 Allergens for tests with known concentrations

2 Cutaneous reactions

Prick Test

3

A Allergen
1   2   3

B

C

D

E

4 Reading of the tests after 20´

Figure 60

In immune complex diseases caused by inhalation, it is important above all to remove the cause of contamination (barns containing mouldy hay should be emptied, hay should be stored after extensive drying, pigeons, parrots, etc. should be removed). Recovery from this type of disease is usually spontaneous, with the exception of ABPA (aspergillosis). The only useful drug may be cortisone. Protracted immune complex diseases may have serious sequelae, such as chronic pulmonary heart failure.

Extrinsic alveolitis sometimes raises difficult problems of differential diagnosis (tuberculosis, sarcoidosis, collagen diseases, etc.). Occurrence of spontaneous pneumothorax may be revealing.

2.9 Skin Tests in Allergy

Skin tests are a practical application of a type I reaction for diagnostic purposes.

The allergologist has at his disposal a series of allergens at known concentrations, contained in easily identifiable bottles (**Figure 60: ❶**). The skin test consists of introducing a minimal amount of allergen into the epidermis or dermis.

There are several test techniques:

– **cutaneous reaction (scratch test)**: consists of simply making a small scratch and placing a drop of allergen solution on it;
– **intradermal reaction**: involves injecting a very small amount of allergen intradermally, using a syringe fitted with a very fine needle (tuberculin syringe);
– **prick test**: consists of depositing a small droplet of allergen on the skin ❸ and puncturing through this droplet using a special needle. This is the most commonly used method.
– finally, the **epidermal test (patch test)** should not be omitted. It consists of placing the test substance on healthy skin under an adhesive occlusive patch. Development of local eczema after 48 hours permits us to identify the cause of contact dermatitis. Epidermal tests can reveal type IV allergies.

Numerous irritant substances provoke urticaria or eczema and do not necessarily cause allergy, e. g., immediate urticaria to stinging nettle or inflammatory reactions to various plants (primulas, tulips, geraniums, fumitory, etc). Some skin reactions are clearly of a toxic nature. For example Dieffenbachia (an indoor plant) releases corrosive oxalates.

In the first three of these tests, reactions are read after 20 minutes. In whatever technique, if the reaction is positive, a small and pruriginous wheal appears within 10–20 minutes, surrounded by an erythematous zone. The wheal, pruritus, and erythema are known as **Lewis' triad**. Wheal pseudopods may appear if the reaction is very violent.

In ❷ are shown five tests carried out on the forearm. Test 2 is strongly positive and test 5 is slightly positive. These tests may be **falsely positive** in patients suffering from dermographism, or if substances known as histamine releasers are introduced into the skin. For this reason, it is required to perform a control test with the diluent used to carry out the tests (negative control), and in parallel with a histamine or codeine phosphate solution (positive control). **False negative** results are also possible, if the patient is under influence of antihistamines or of other drugs with an antihistaminic effect (e. g., ketotifen, or certain tricyclic antidepressants).

Antihistamines should be avoided for at least three days before the tests and up to four weeks before in the case of astemizole. In contrast, corticosteroids and beta-mimetics do not interfere with the reactions.

The allergens used should be well known, otherwise there is a danger of provoking very violent reactions and even anaphylactic shock, which could lead to death.

Allergens most commonly used for skin tests include:

– **House dust mites**, especially Dermatophagoides pteronyssinus and Dermatophagoides farinae (the latter mainly in Japan and the USA). Storage mites (Glyciphagus, Tyrophagus, Myacerus Centneri, etc.), capable of causing respiratory symptoms in cereal handlers and farmers, should also be mentioned.
– **Pollens**, especially pollens of graminaceae, plantain, Compositae such as artemisia, and tree pollens such as birch and hazel. Pollens also vary from one region to another. Thus, in the USA, ragweed or ambrosia plays a major part in allergology, while allergy to pellitory and olive trees is very common in southern Europe but is virtually unknown elsewhere.
– **Flour**, used in bakeries and related trades. Allergy to flour may allow some patients to receive compensation on the grounds that they have an occupational disease.
– **Animal hair and skin dander**, particularly cats and dogs (the allergy may be to only one breed of dog), guinea-pigs, rabbits, and hamsters, and hair of farm animals, such as horses, pigs and cows. Roe-deer, antelopes, and hares may cause allergies in hunters and in cooks.
– **Moulds**: the problem of moulds is more complicated, since there are almost 100,000 known mould species. The main moulds used in allergology are Alternaria, Aspergillus, Cladosporium, and Penicillium, but their extracts are rarely pure and there are numerous cross-reactions between different species.
– **Hymenoptera venoms**: tests with these allergens should be performed with utmost caution, in view of the risk of anaphylactic shock which they may produce, and the poor stability of diluted allergen solutions. It is preferable to use RAST or CAST.
– **Food allergens** are often disappointing in practice, either because the extract itself does not contain the required allergens (some food allergens are rather unstable and are only present in raw and fresh food) or because digestive allergy is not always accompanied by a corresponding skin allergy. Their use, and especially their interpretation, should be reserved for physicians specialized in this field.

2.10 Hyposensitization – Immunotherapy

Allergy to certain antigens lends itself particularly well to specific **immunotherapy**. Immunotherapy is often called desensitization therapy, which is not a correct term, because the patient is not desensitized but simply made *less* sensitive to the allergen. Immunotherapy induces in fact **hyposensitization**. The principle underlying immunotherapy is to inject the allergic patient with increasing doses of allergen. This technique responds to precise rules. Poorly selected doses of vaccine may give rise to local reactions (edema at the site of injection), syndromes (rhinitis, asthma), or even systemic reactions (urticaria and even anaphylactic shock). **Emergency treatment for anaphylactic shock is adrenaline**.

The efficacy of immunotherapy has been confirmed in correctly conducted studies (double-blind, placebo controlled) for only a limited number of allergens: house dust mites, grass pollens, birch, mountain cedar, ragweed (ambrosia), cat and dog allergens, and several rarer moulds (Alternaria and Cladosporium).

Some allergen vaccines are very efficient (house dust mites, pollens), while others are less so, but may nevertheless be useful (animal dander). Still others are relatively effective but dangerous, such as with certain moulds (either because they cause formation of precipitins, e.g., Aspergillus, or because of frequent adverse reactions, as e.g., in immunotherapy to Alternaria or Cladosporium). Patients are usually allergic to only a few allergens. No one is ever "allergic to everything." The choice and composition of the allergen vaccine should be based above all on the patient's history and on the results of skin tests, and to a lesser degree on the results of serologic tests to detect specific IgE, such as RAST, and others. When in doubt, provocation tests or mediator release tests should be used. Before the onset of immunotherapy, eviction of the responsible allergens should be attempted. Only allergens playing a major role are to be incorporated in the vaccine and never more than two (rarely three) allergen vaccines should be used simultaneously in the same patient. It is unwise to put several allergens in the same bottle, because, in case of an adverse reaction, it would be embarrassingly impossible to determine the allergen responsible, and equally impossible to reduce selectively the dose of this allergen. Furthermore, some allergens seem to exert a proteolytic effect on other allergens present in the same bottle.

It is not entirely clear why hyposensitization works. A popular theory, which was convincing for a long time, has recently become less probable. It concerns the appearance of specific non-allergy-inducing IgG (e.g., IgG4) which competes with allergy-inducing IgE: these are called **"blocking antibodies."** This hypothesis implies that non-cytophilic IgG 4 neutralize allergens before these come into contact with IgE, thereby preventing the degranulation of mast cells.

According to more recent views, allergen injection favors the production of Ts lymphocytes (suppressors) and especially **Th1 lymphocytes** at the expense of **Th2 lymphocytes**. The range of produced lymphokines shifts to the disadvantage of pro-inflammatory lymphokines (IL-4, IL-3, IL-5). This, on the one hand, prevents maturation of certain B lymphocytes with a corresponding decrease of IgE-secreting plasma cells. On the other hand, it decreases mediator release by the inflammatory cells involved (eosinophils, mast cells, basophils).

These mechanisms do not, however, explain the efficacy of accelerated ("rush") immunotherapy, where the progressive (but not explosive) exhaustion of mast cell granules, released in small quantities after each injection of vaccine, is believed, among others, to be responsible.

Immunotherapy appears to act on the late phase of asthma, rather than on the early phase, by affecting T lymphocytes, among others. Many studies are currently in progress to determine the exact mechanism of hyposensitization and the possibility of blocking harmful IgE by methods other than immunotherapy with allergens (e.g., anti-IgE or anti-idiotype antibodies).

Meanwhile the classical immunotherapy method is still used, but at present with the assistance of much higher quality allergen vaccines. One of these advances is the use of depot preparations, i.e., allergens which are absorbed slowly, minimizing thereby the risk of overdosage and permitting injection of much higher allergen doses at intervals of perhaps one injection per month (maintenance therapy). One of the possibilities to prepare depot vaccines is to adsorb allergens to aluminum hydroxide gel.

Chemically modified **("allergoids")** or polymerized allergens are also increasingly used.

With respect to the age at which immunotherapy can be started: in practice, children can be hyposensitized from the age of two years and even 18 months on, i.e., as soon as a responsible allergen can be identified. It should, however, be noted that most of the time skin and RAST tests become positive only after the age of 2–3 years; therefore, it is often difficult to know against which allergen younger children are allergic. The decision to vaccinate such young children depends on the severity of symptoms, familial history of allergic antecedents, motivation, and the psychological context, as well as the results of studies currently under way to determine whether immunotherapy carried out very early may reduce allergies in older children and adults.

Oral or sublingual immunotherapy, instead of immunotherapy by injection, is still controversial, regarding its efficacy and its mechanism(s), although an number of recent studies have cast this approach in an increasingly favorable light.

2.11 Outline of Therapy for Type I Allergies

In the framework of this Atlas, it is not possible to mention the many finer points and subtleties of anti-allergy treatments, but we can introduce a number of the key elements involved.

Accurate diagnostic investigations before any therapy is the key to success. It is essential to assess that an allergy is indeed present and to attempt identification of the responsible allergen(s). The patient's history is of prime importance: it should be detailed, and taking it accurately requires experience. Indeed, this process can resemble a police investigation. Psychological factors may be fundamental in both adults and children.

Once an allergen is suspected, **skin tests** should be carried out, and possibly some **serological tests**, although only a limited number of allergens may be investigated by these methods. A first serological screening may also be performed. Various additional examinations are occasionally required: chest or sinus X-rays, lung function tests, cellular tests and various analyses.

The first and most important therapeutic step is **eviction of the harmful allergen**, whenever possible. This is not always easy – like separation from a favorite dog or cat – and not always possible, as in the case of allergy to pollens. Exclusion of allergens may be effective in allergy to house dust, provoked mainly by Dermatophagoides mites, but it requires a lot of energy: removal of carpets and wall-to-wall carpets, use of synthetic bed linen with regular vacuuming of mattresses, covering of mattresses, pillows and bedspreads with impermeable covers, acaricide sprays (fortunately, aerosol cans are gradually disappearing from the market due to the ecological damage caused by propellent gases which they contain), and replacement of old mattresses. Test strips are also marketed in some countries (Acarex test®), which yield some idea of the density of house dust mites in a mattress or in other domestic textiles. This test is based on the demonstration of guanine excreted by the mites. There is a fairly precise correlation between mite activity and guanine content in an environment. Likewise, it has become possible to detect allergens in house dust through immunological tests, such as Dustcreen®.

Immunotherapy may be an effective therapeutic approach, depending on the incriminating allergen(s) detected, and on the severity of the allergy involved.

In addition to these specific treatments a **symptomatic therapy** is often well advised. Asthma is presently considered above all as a chronic inflammatory disease and is no longer seen as a pathology merely characterized by episodes of bronchospasm. This inflammatory state of the airways may even be present in asymptomatic patients. Accordingly, much weight is given nowadays to **local corticosteroids** applied by inhalation with a nebulizer (beclomethasone, budesonide). If severe bronchospasm attacks appear despite corticosteroids, **Beta-mimetic bronchodilators** remain indicated. These can reduce symptoms but do not cure asthma. The use of spacer chambers for the inhalation of drugs, such as corticosteroids and betamimetics, markedly increases their efficacy. Good cooperation with the patient is essential, particularly regarding the use of an individual peak flow meter. The use of local corticosteroids must be prolonged and requires hormonal controls.

Theophylline is still widely used, but its bronchodilating action is weak, and its therapeutic index is narrow (headache, vomiting, nausea, excessive nervousness, etc. are not uncommon, especially in children). Therefore, it requires tedious blood control determinations (threshold not to be exceeded: $10–20\,\mu g/ml$). Theophylline potentiates possible side effects of beta-mimetics (tachycardia, tremor). The combination of theophylline with beta-mimetics does not seem to increase the efficacy of both substances.

Ipratropium and its derivatives in aerosol form exert selective vagolytic action on the bronchi and may be very effective in some asthmatic patients.

The various allergic syndromes are sometimes treated with oral and even injectable corticosteroids in cases of severe inflammation, but only following very strict guidelines. **Disodium cromoglycate** (DSCG) is used as an effective prophylactic drug (with a Halermatic or Spinhaler inhaler, or in aerosol form). It is also used in solution for local application in the eyes and nose. An oral form is available in certain countries. One of its derivatives, **nedocromil**, is efficacious and adds to the effects of DSCG a marked anti-inflammatory action, often allowing reduction of corticosteroid doses. Certain drugs permitting reduction of corticosteroid doses (steroid-sparing-drugs) which treat corticosteroid-resistant cases are currently under study: these are essentially methotrexate, but also chloroquine, dapsone and cyclosporin or related drugs.

The drug Ketotifen possesses actions similar to those of antihistamines, but it is not always well tolerated, sometimes producing drowsiness, and even bulimia. Opinions about its prophylactic value, particularly in children, are rather divided.

Antihistamines are especially useful in rhinitis, conjunctivitis, and in all types of pruriginous lesions. Some among them may also be effective in asthma (cetirizine) by inhibiting the influx of eosinophils.

Antibiotics are prescribed in cases of superinfection, which may be more frequent than imagined.

Intelligent **psychotherapy** may be of great value, especially in allergic patients, who are often overanxious.

Part Three

Elements of Immune Pathology

3.1 Immunoglobulin Diseases

The pathological increase of immunoglobulins is due to an abnormal proliferation of plasmocytes. This increase may affect all the immunoglobulins **(polyclonal gammopathy)** or just one class of Ig **(monoclonal gammopathy)**. An Ig present in abnormal amounts is called a **paraprotein**. Such a protein can clearly be seen on serum electrophoresis plates, where it appears as a band in the gamma zone.

About 1% of the population has benign monoclonal gammopathy. In these cases, long-term follow-up is required, in view of possible clonal proliferation of B lymphocytes.

Simple antigenic stimulation may increase the concentration of immunoglobulins. The first to increase is IgM, followed by IgG **(Figure 28)**. An abnormal increase of immunoglobulins occurs in many chronic disorders: such as sarcoidosis, tuberculosis, collagenoses, liver cirrhosis, etc. Synthesis of a single class of immunoglobulins or even a

single chain of immunoglobulins accompanies some immunoproliferative diseases. Such diseases are known as **monoclonal gammopathies.** They include myelomas, Waldenström's macroglobulinemia, heavy-chain disease, and light chain disease.

Substances known as **cryoglobulins** are present in some disorders and in some elderly people: they precipitate in vitro at +4°C (in patients possessing such cryoglobulins, a contact test with an ice cube provokes local edema very fast). If body temperature decreases, vascular obstruction accompanied by edema, ischemia, and ulceration may occur, due to these cryoglobulins. Cryoglobulins are encountered in mononucleosis, myelomas, Waldenström's disease, and occasionally in patients with no detectable disorder.

3.2 Immune Deficiencies

Aside from gammopathies, immune deficiencies may affect either humoral or cellular immunity or both. Occasionally the phenomena overlap, or may be accompanied by some deficit of complement or of blood cell phagocytosis.

3.2.1 Humoral immune deficiencies

Of course, these disorders cause an increased susceptibility to bacterial infections. A baby born with its mother's IgG may suffer physiological delay in producing its own Ig (see **Figure 28**). Thus, there will be a fairly short critical period during which the baby is very vulnerable: at the time it has eliminated maternal Ig, but has not yet produced its own Ig. Serious immune deficiencies include **Bruton's disease**, characterized by an absence of B lymphocytes and agammaglobulinaemia.

Acquired agammaglobulinemias exist mainly in neoplasms, with invasion and destruction of lymphoid tissues.

Dysgammaglobulinemias result from defective synthesis of one or other type of Ig. The best known disease of this kind is **ataxia-telangiectasia** (major IgA deficiency, cerebral atrophy and telangiectasia).

Wiskott-Aldrich syndrome is characterized by IgM de-

ficiency, increased IgG and IgE, eczema, asthma, repeated infections, thrombocytopenia and T-lymphocyte deficiency.

Isolated IgA deficiency, occasionally associated with elevated IgE levels, is remarkably common, and occurs in about 1 out of every 700 persons.

Deficiency of IgG subclasses, especially IgG2, is frequently associated with recurrent respiratory tract infections in childhood, and is treated by the injection of immunoglobulins.

3.2.2 Cellular immune deficiencies

This deficiency causes high vulnerability to gram-negative bacteria, viruses, mycoses, mycobacteria, and even to BCG.

It may be related to hereditary thymus insufficiency, as in **Nezelof's syndrome**, with thymus atrophy but normal Ig levels, and in **DiGeorge's syndrome**, in which the thymus is absent, but with normal Ig levels.

However, cellular immune deficiencies are more frequently acquired and appear following immunosuppressive treatment or infection by the human immunodeficiency virus (HIV), which is responsible for the acquired immunodeficiency syndrome **(AIDS)**. The HIV virus has a special affinity for Th (CD4) lymphocytes, in which it multiplies until destroying them. Infections most frequently encountered during the course of the disease, known as "opportunistic infections," include: Pneumocystis carinii pneumonia, Toxoplasma brain abscess, atypical mycobacterial infection and tuberculosis, herpetic infections (herpes simplex and zona), and Cryptococcus meningitis. The disease is accompanied by absolute lymphopenia and often by considerable polyclonal hypergammaglobulinemia. Kaposi's sarcoma also frequently appears in AIDS. It especially affects the skin and intestine.

A decrease in cellular immmunity, particularly of type IV skin reactions to bacterial and parasitic antigens, is the most frequent immunological change observed in **aging.** It explains the lessened resistance of aging individuals to infections, to cancer, and their tendency to develop auto-immune diseases.

3.2.3 Mixed deficiencies

Mixed deficiency involves both humoral and cellular deficiency. It causes **Swiss-type agammaglobulinaemia** or **thymolymphoplasia**, and ends in early death.

Immune deficiencies, which are sometimes only temporary, can often be caused by cancerous disorders, leukemias, Hodgkin's disease, infectious mononucleosis, certain infections such as leprosy and tuberculosis, viral diseases, common measles, and certainly also malnutrition.

3.2.4. Non-specific deficiencies

In addition to humoral and cellular immune deficiencies, there are various non-specific deficiencies, which affect **neutrophils.** These may include: reduction or complete absence of neutrophils, anomalies in their bactericidal and phagocytic functions, and/or chemotactic disorders. Some of these disorders may be linked to the use of certain drugs, such as Levamisole. In addition to neutrophil disorders, there may be a **complement deficiency**, the most common form being a deficit of C1s esterase inhibitor, causing hereditary angioneurotic edema.

A. STRUCTURE OF HIV VIRUS

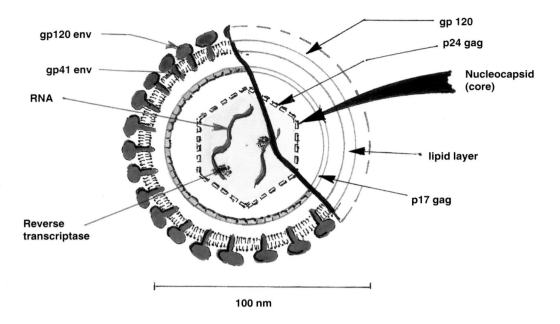

gp120 env

gp41 env

RNA

Reverse
transcriptase

gp 120

p24 gag

Nucleocapsid
(core)

lipid layer

p17 gag

100 nm

B. LIFE CYCLE OF HIV VIRUS

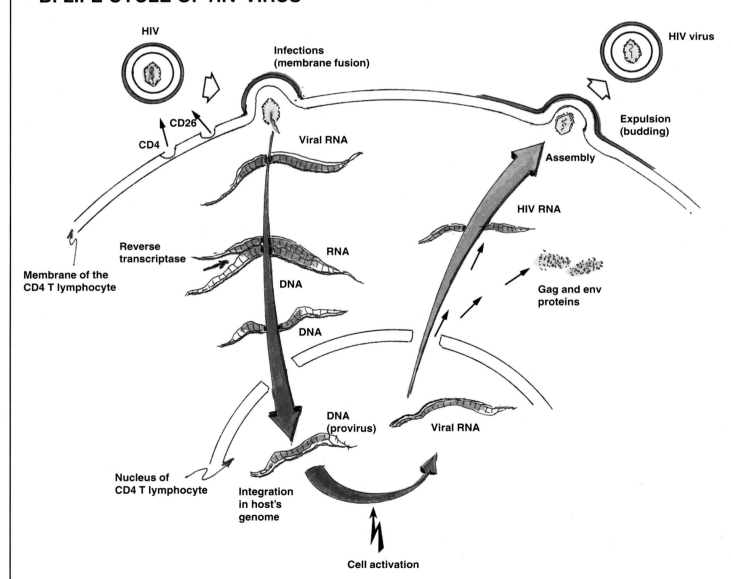

HIV

Infections
(membrane fusion)

HIV virus

CD26

CD4

Viral RNA

Expulsion
(budding)

Assembly

Membrane of the
CD4 T lymphocyte

Reverse
transcriptase

RNA

DNA

HIV RNA

Gag and env
proteins

DNA

Nucleus of
CD4 T lymphocyte

DNA
(provirus)

Integration
in host's
genome

Viral RNA

Cell activation

Figure 61

3.3 Acquired Immunodeficiency Syndrome: AIDS

AIDS is an immune deficiency syndrome resulting from infection by the HIV virus, which may be transmitted by sexual intercourse, by prenatal or perinatal relationship between mother and child, or by contact with contaminated blood or blood products.

Acute primary HIV infection manifests sometimes as pseudo-influenza syndrome with fever and skin rash, but is most often clinically silent. First symptoms, which may take years to become apparent, usually consist of polyadenopathy, weight loss, nocturnal sweating and possibly oral infection with Candida albicans ("trush"). When immune deficiency has become more severe, the complete pattern of AIDS becomes manifest, particularly in form of **"opportunistic" infections,** so called, because they are due to pathogenic germs against which the organism usually defends itself efficiently. Pulmonary infections due to Pneumocystis carinii or to various secondary species of mycobacteria (avian, bovine) are rather frequent.

Likewise, certain types of tumors, like **Kaposi's sarcoma** or **Burkitt's lymphoma** are frequently also involved. Once the AIDS syndrome is fully developed, the evolution is practically always lethal. This must not be necessarily the case for the HIV infection itself. Indeed, most recent statistics show that with good hygiene and optimal medical supervision, almost half of HIV positive individuals have not developed AIDS after 10 years of infection.

This shows that certain factors related to the infection itself (e. g., more or less virulent HIV strain), to the infected individual (e. g., immunological anti-HIV response) or other independent factors (e. g., general hygiene, other venereal diseases and associated infections, quality of nutrition, etc.) may influence the clinical evolution. However, it is scientifically unjustified to conclude that the association of these various secondary factors is the cause of AIDS, as some still pretend.

Certainly, there are numerous causes of acquired immune deficiency which may cause the one or the other similar symptom, but only HIV infection brings about the characteristic full clinical picture of AIDS, with its accompanying immunological and physiopathological abnormalities, such as a decrease in T lymphocytes of the CD4 class.

The HIV virus is an RNA virus (called a retrovirus, because it incorporates into the DNA genome of the host) and it has a relatively complex structure, as suggested in **Figure 61, A.** The most important constituents are
- the nucleus containing the genome,
- the encompassing isolated RNA chains,
- the enzyme "reverse transcriptase" or RNA polymerase and
- capside proteins (determined by genes called "gag"). The main gag proteins are denominated p24 and p17.

The viral nucleus is surrounded by an envelope formed by a lipidic layer, and in this envelope proteins deriving from "env" genes are inserted. The most important env protein is called gp160 and it splits into two fragments, gp120 and gp41.

The HIV virus has a particular attraction for human cells possessing the CD4, and more recently also the CD26 receptor on their surface. These receptors bind the gp120 virus protein **(Figure 61, B).** Such cells are above all CD4 T lymphocytes, but include also certain monocyte or macrophage lines, such as Langerhans and dendritic cells. Fixation of a viral HIV particle on the cell membrane is followed by fusion of viral and cell membranes, induced by gp41, releasing free RNA chains inside the cell.

Reverse transcriptase may then fulfill its role, which is, on the basis of RNA chains, to produce the corresponding DNA chains characteristic of the HIV virus. Those DNA chains integrate into the host's genome, where they may remain resting in a state of "provirus" for many years. Following cell activation, however, the viral DNA portion may again be transcribed in the reverse sense and generate new RNA HIV chains. These RNA chains will, on the one hand, generate the various viral gag and env proteins, and, on the other hand, assemble into new nuclear capsides which are finally expelled by the host cell.

The immune response to HIV infection is complex. Antibody formation, in particular against gp120, gp41 and p24 proteins, becomes manifest about two to three months after the initial infection **(seroconversion).** Some of the antibodies produced may have protecting and neutralizing effects. However, the fact that the virus attaches with predilection to CD4 T lymphocytes, which are indispensable helper lymphocytes for a normal immune response, will sooner or later lead to severe consequences. The mechanisms by which the HIV virus induces a progressive decrease of CD4 T lymphocytes and paralysis or immune responses are still very controversial, despite intensive research. It is clear that HIV infection does not only affect CD4 cells directly but also indirectly influences several other sections of the immune defense **(Figure 62 A).** The complexity of the reactions in question and the subtlety with which the virus may evade immunological defenses are the main reasons why initial optimism concerning HIV vaccination has turned into some pessimism. Indeed, the raising of an immune response against isolated virus constituents (e. g., gp120) or against killed HIV virus have been shown to be not very efficacious, or even under some circumstances to have a non-protective, facilitating effect on a subsequent HIV infection. The relative pessimism prevailing today seems the more justified in that HIV is not a single virus strain but encompasses numerous more or less pathogenic mutants, somewhat like the influenza virus.

INFECTION

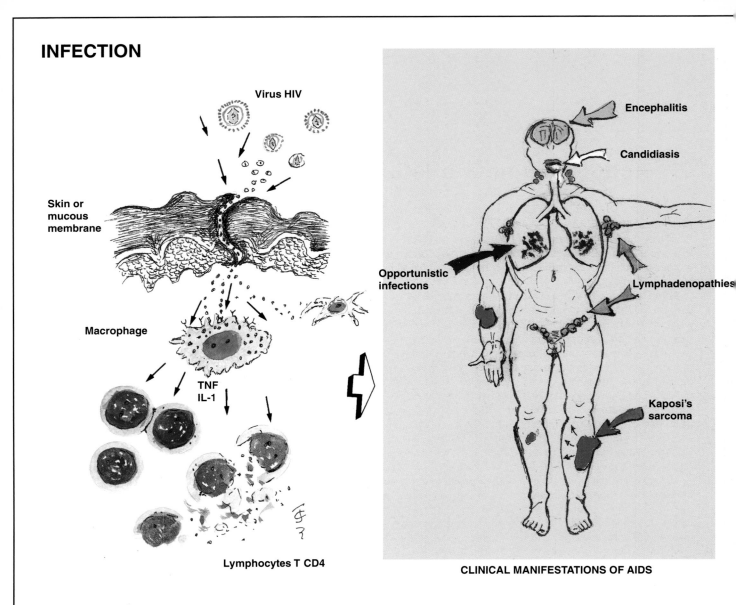

Virus HIV

Skin or mucous membrane

Macrophage

TNF IL-1

Lymphocytes T CD4

Encephalitis

Candidiasis

Opportunistic infections

Lymphadenopathies

Kaposi's sarcoma

CLINICAL MANIFESTATIONS OF AIDS

IMMUNOLOGICAL EVOLUTION OF AIDS

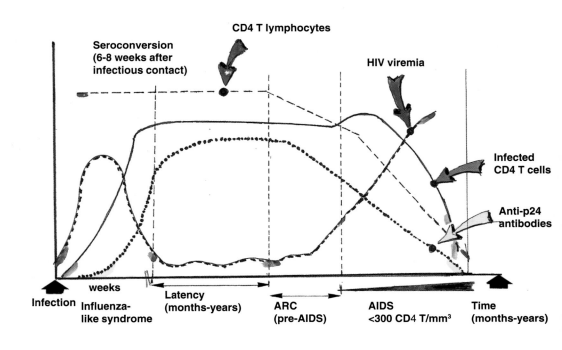

CD4 T lymphocytes

Seroconversion (6-8 weeks after infectious contact)

HIV viremia

Infected CD4 T cells

Anti-p24 antibodies

Infection

weeks

Influenza-like syndrome

Latency (months-years)

ARC (pre-AIDS)

AIDS <300 CD4 T/mm³

Time (months-years)

Figure 62A

Drug therapeutic trials (e. g., with azidothymidine (AZT) blocking action of the reverse transcriptase) are currently based on producing a blockade of enzymatic or transcription processes required for virus replication. Genetic approaches dealing with the complex processes of HIV RNA/DNA transcription are likewise under way.

Figure 62: Destruction of the immune system by the HIV virus

Pathway of infection. The HIV virus infected cells penetrate through skin or mucous lesions ❶ infecting dendritic cells, Langerhans cells and other cells of macrophage lineage ❷. Those cells are not killed by viral replication and serve as reservoir and transport agents for the virus. The virus may likewise infect whatever CD4 T lymphocytes they encounter.

Dissemination and evolution of infection (Figure 62, A):
The HIV virus initially infects lymph nodes (polyadenopathy) and the central nervous system. Due to the immune deficiency provoked by HIV infection, opportunistic infections (i. e., infection provoked by usually non-pathogenic microorganisms) become manifest, particularly in the mouth ("thrush": candidiasis) and in lungs (e. g., Pneumocystis carinii pneumonia). Likewise, lymphoid and skin tumors frequently develop (Kaposi's sarcoma).

From an immunological point of view, an initial period of viremia manifested by an influenza-like syndrome is followed by a more or less prolonged silent period, during which the only manifestation of infection is the appearance of antibodies, particularly directed against envelope antigens such as gp120 and gp41. Then, during clinical evolution towards a **pre-AIDS** stage (**ARC**: AIDS-related complex) and towards manifest **AIDS**, we observe a progressive decrease of CD4 T lymphocytes and renewed increase in viremia, associated with a decrease or apparent disappearance of anti-gp24 antibodies, complexed to the excess of viral antigens in circulation.

MECHANISMS OF DESTRUCTION OF IMMUNE APPARATUS BY THE HIV VIRUS

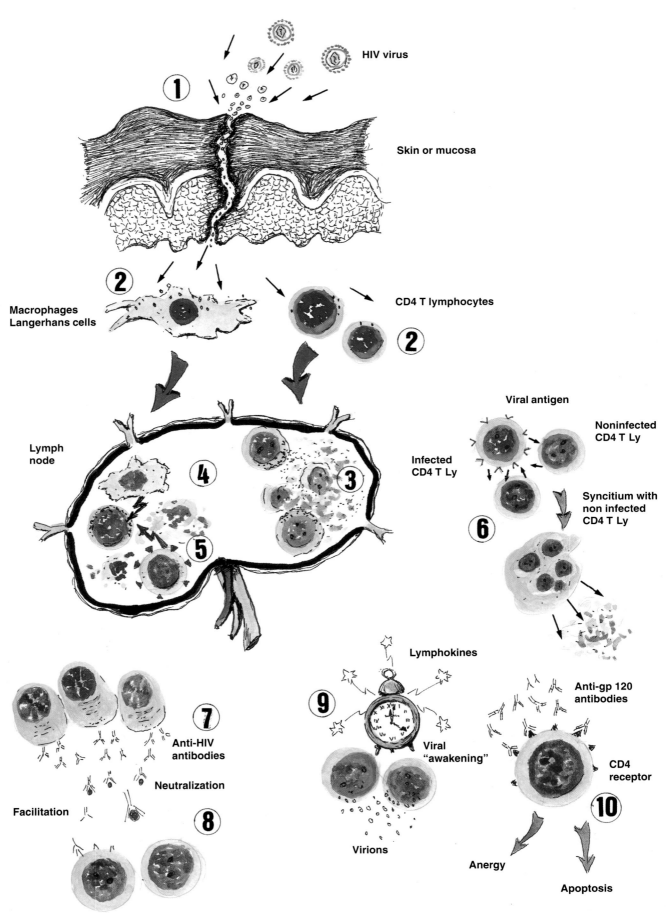

Figure 62B

Main mechanisms responsible for the immune deficiency (Figure 62, B): Following transmucosal or transcutaneous invasion by HIV viruses ❶ and their penetration in macrophages and T lymphocytes ❷, various direct or indirect mechanisms contribute to the decrease of CD4 T helper lymphocytes. These are in particular: ❸ cytopathogenic effects of viral replication causing cell budding; ❹ destruction of T lymphocytes by activated macrophages or by ❺ cytotoxic T lymphocytes specific for some HIV antigens (e. g., gp120-derived peptides).

The interaction between T lymphocytes expressing viral antigens ❻ and CD4 T lymphocytes may lead to the formation and destruction of giant cells (syncitia).

Antibody formation against HIV antigens ❼ may have a virus neutralizing effect, but may also facilitate cellular infection by forming HIV-antibody complexes ❽. Various non-specific stimulations (e. g., lymphokines) may favor the awakening of the virus hitherto at rest in an infected T lymphocyte and cause accelerated viral replication ❾. Finally, interaction of anti-gp120 antibodies or soluble gp120 antigen with CD4 cellular receptors ❿ may cause paralysis of cellular functions (anergy) or slow programmed cell death (apoptosis).

Various non-specific elements accompanying the viral infection, such as the production of suppressor lymphokines (e. g., TNF-β, interferon γ) by infected macrophages ❷, polygammaglobulinemia and relative stimulation of CD8 T lymphocytes, may contribute, in addition to the destruction of CD4 T lymphocytes, to the progressive immune deficiency which is typical for AIDS.

RENAL IMMUNOPATHOLOGY: MECHANISMS

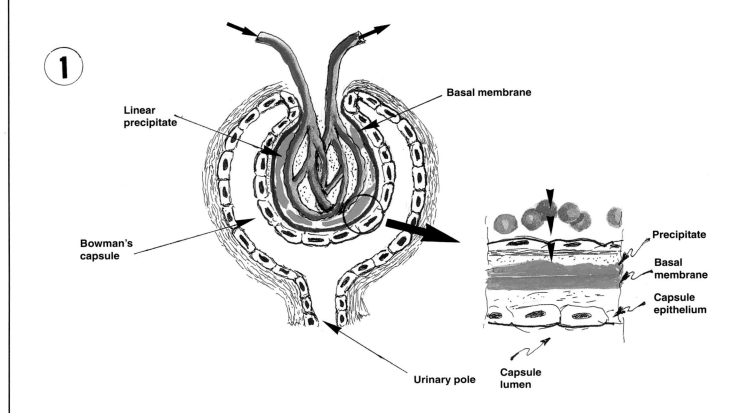

1

Basal membrane

Linear precipitate

Bowman's capsule

Urinary pole

Precipitate

Basal membrane

Capsule epithelium

Capsule lumen

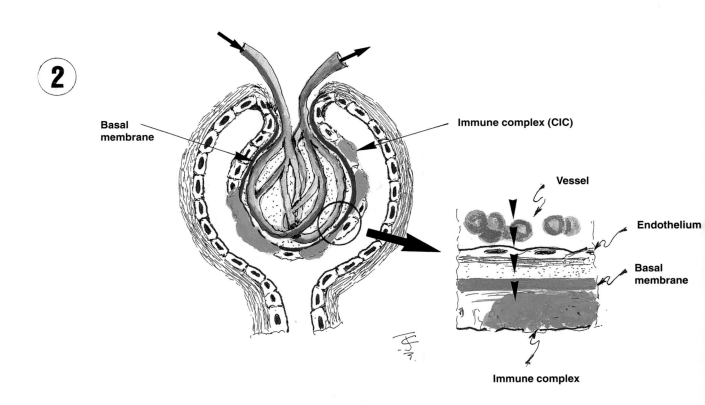

2

Basal membrane

Immune complex (CIC)

Vessel

Endothelium

Basal membrane

Immune complex

Figure 63

3.4 Renal Immunopathology

Kidney disorders during immunological diseases are very frequent, either because the kidneys themselves are the target organ **(Goodpasture's syndrome)**, or because the renal filter retains immunological debris capable of provoking autoimmune reactions.

Experimentally, if an animal is injected with kidney extracts, it develops antibodies directed against kidneys and a linear precipitate appears on the basal membrane: after passing through the vascular endothelium, an antibasal membrane antibody is fixed to the basal membrane. Such an experimental nephritis is known as **Masugi nephritis (Figure 63 ❶)**.

Common mechanisms in the majority of glomerulonephritis (GN) diseases with some immune component involve immune complexes (IC) **(Figure 63 ❷)**. These are either circulating IC (CIC), retained by the renal filter, or they are IC due to antigens "inserted" in the basal membrane

and inducing local fixation of antibodies of varying specificity. In most cases, the presence of such IC causes activation of complement, which triggers a cascade of reactions leading to destruction of the affected glomerulus. Biological tests may to varying degrees demonstrate CIC, hypocomplementemia, and antinuclear antibodies (ANA).

Some examples. Berger's disease is characterized by deposits of IgA in the mesangium of glomeruli, where special CIC (formed by IgA and fibronectin) can be detected. In **lupus glomerulonephritis**, there seems to be a cause-effect relationship between the presence of anti-DNA antibodies, DNA-anti-DNA IC, and nephropathy. In **Goodpasture's syndrome,** specific glomerular and pulmonary anti-basal membrane antibodies are found. Tubular anti-basal membrane antibodies are also found in certain forms of interstitial tubular nephritis, particularly when induced by drugs.

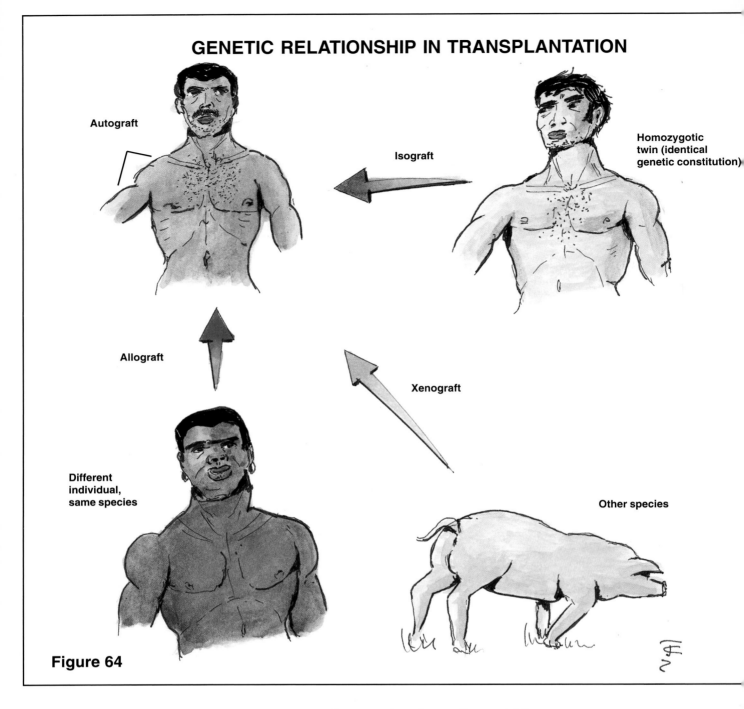

GENETIC RELATIONSHIP IN TRANSPLANTATION

Autograft

Isograft

Homozygotic twin (identical genetic constitution)

Allograft

Xenograft

Different individual, same species

Other species

Figure 64

3.5 Organ Transplantation: Rejection Phenomenon

Transplantation immunology is getting increasingly important, from a clinical point of view, now involving cellular grafts (for example, blood transfusion and bone marrow grafts), as well as organ transplants (kidney, heart, liver, pancreas, lungs, cornea, skin, etc.). In addition, individual cellular antigens determining tissular compatibility or incompatibility **("histocompatibility")** play an important role in immunobiology, as they participate in immune recognition and antigen presentation phenomena.

The immunological barrier to transplantation is determined by genetic differences between donor and receiver **(Figure 64).** While this barrier may not exist when donor and receiver are the same individual **(autograft)** or individ-

uals of identical genetic constitution **(isograft),** it may become quite important when the donor is a different individual from the same species **(allograft)** or from another species **(xenograft).**

The immunological barrier is essentially due to **histocompatibility antigens** present on numerous cell membranes. These antigens are part of several systems, such as the **ABO system** and **Rhesus system**, better known from problems of compatibility in blood transfusion, and the **HLA system** ("Human Leukocyte Antigens"). The latter constitutes the **Major Histocompatibility Complex (MHC)** in mammals and rodents.

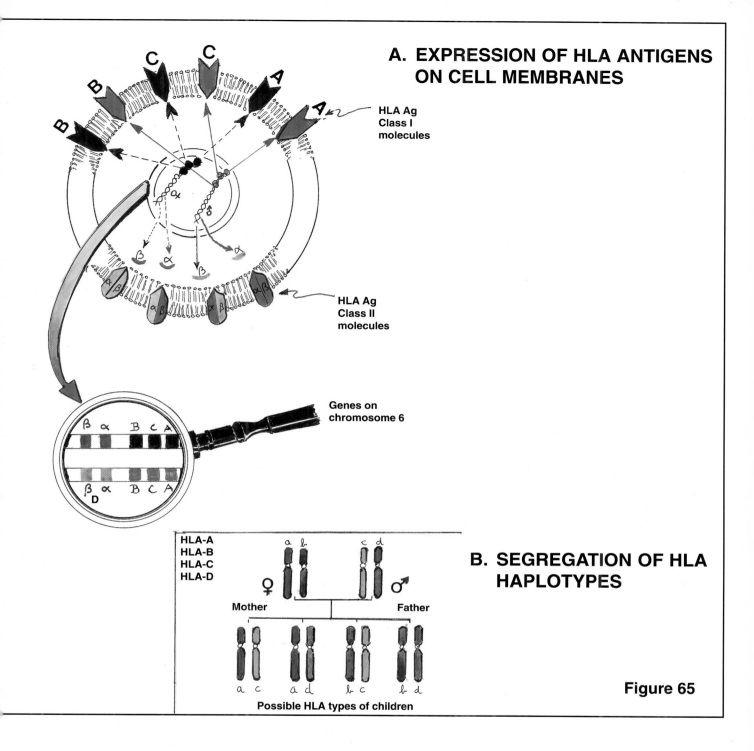

A. EXPRESSION OF HLA ANTIGENS ON CELL MEMBRANES

HLA Ag
Class I
molecules

HLA Ag
Class II
molecules

Genes on
chromosome 6

B. SEGREGATION OF HLA HAPLOTYPES

HLA-A
HLA-B
HLA-C
HLA-D

♀ Mother   Father ♂

Possible HLA types of children

Figure 65

The **HLA system** consists of membrane proteins, divided in two classes: **Class I MHC antigens**, expressed as one single polypeptide chain and dependent on three genetic loci A, B, and D **(Figure 65, A)**, and **Class II MHC antigens**, consisting of two chains: A and B. Class II antigens stem from genes belonging to locus D, which is situated, like loci A, B, and C, on the short arm of chromosome 6 in man **(Figure 65, B)**.

Class I antigens are present on most nucleated cells, while the distribution of class II antigens is more limited, in particular to cells capable of presenting antigens (dendritic cells, macrophages, B cells, activated T cells or endothelial cells). Class I and Class II antigens are also different in func-

tional terms: class II antigens participate in the recognition of antigens presented to CD4 T helper lymphocytes **(Figure 21)**, while class II antigens are recognized by CD8 T lymphocytes acting as suppressor or cytotoxic lymphocytes.

Histocompatibility antigens are expressed co-dominantly on cells, i. e., the presence of a gene corresponding to loci A, B, C, or D deriving from father and mother leads to expression on the cell membrane of the corresponding antigens **(Figure 65, A)**. Genes of loci A, B, C and D are usually inherited globally, as haplotype a or b (from the mother) and c or d (from the father) **(Figure 65, B)**. Therefore, there may be in principle four types of children. It is possible, even

125

IMMUNOLOGICAL MECHANISMS OF TRANSPLANT REJECTION

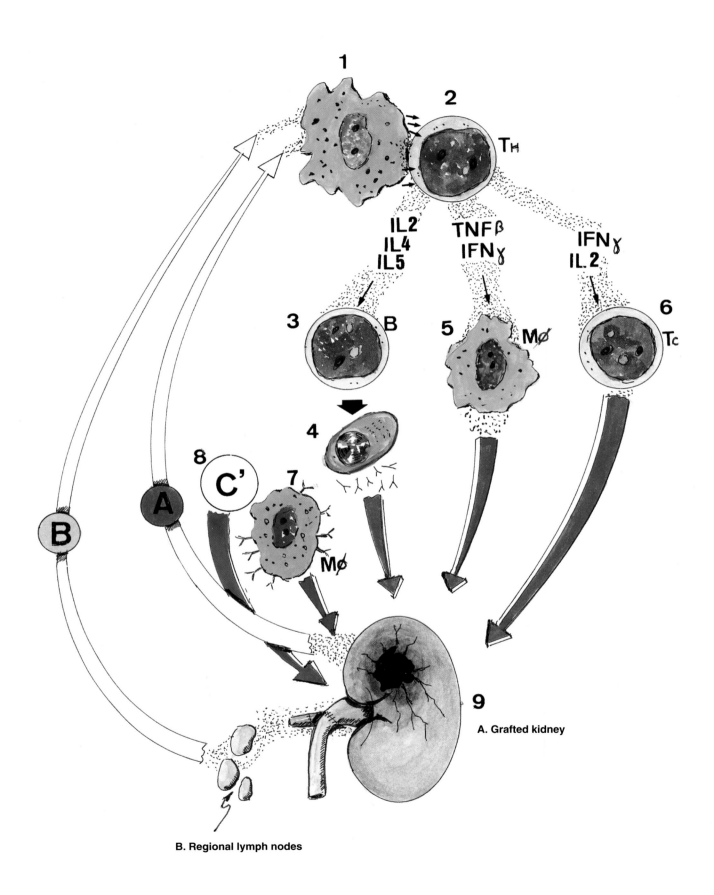

A. Grafted kidney

B. Regional lymph nodes

Figure 66

among children who are not homozygotic twins, to encounter a brother or a sister with an identical HLA formula. As a result, we are always interested in looking for an HLA identical donor in the patient's own family, in case of transplantation or especially where repeated blood transfusions are involved. In contrast, as there are about 80 known allelic genes for loci A, B and C and 35 for locus D, the chances of finding an HLA identical non-related donor are relatively slim.

Transplantation between a donor and receiver which are not identical for their histocompatibility antigens, leads obligatorily to **immunological rejection**, if the immune system of the receiver is intact. T lymphocytes are mainly responsible for this phenomenon, as suggested in **Figure 66**.

However, the rejection mechanism is quite complicated. It may involve recognition of MHC antigens directly encountered in the graft **(A)** or as antigens reaching regional lymph nodes **(B)**. Class II MHC antigens presented by accessory cells ❶ stimulate CD4 T helper lymphocytes ❷ while recognition of class I antigens stimulate CD8 T cytotoxic lymphocytes ❹. These lymphocytes play an important role in primary and chronic rejection reactions. Production of various cytokines by activated lymphocytes will amplify and trigger additional phenomena, such as activation of cytotoxic macrophages ❺, stimulation of B lymphocytes ❸ and production of antibodies against MHC antigens ❻. These antibodies may then "arm" cytotoxic cells (ADCC; **Figure 66** ❼) or directly attack endothelial cells

with intervention of complement ❽. All these mechanisms lead to rejection of the transplanted organ ❾. Anti-MHC antibodies are in particular responsible for hyperacute rejection, such as occur in a second transplantation after rejection of the first one.

Of course, somehow preventing a rejection is essential for successful transplantation. A first step consists in reducing as much as possible the MHC differences between donor and receiver, which is possible in elective transplantation (e. g., kidney) by setting up organ banks and receiver networks for potential organ donors. It is likewise possible, in a **non-specific** manner to minimize rejection, using drugs suppressing cellular activation (corticosteroids), cytokine production (cyclosporin) or cellular proliferation (azathioprine). However, more **specific** interventions are the subject of intense studies, with the purpose of avoiding the frequent side effects of immunosuppressive drugs. Induction of immunological tolerance by administration of antigens from the graft during embryonal development of the receiver, although possible in immunological experiments is obviously impractical in clinical situations. Yet, the administration of histocompatibility antigens, or their corresponding antibodies in adults, under certain conditions, permits the attenuation of rejection **(facilitation phenomenon).**

Attempts to introduce human MHC antigens into animal species, such as pigs, by transgenic technology (introduction of genes from one individual or one species to another), are currently under way. This would enable us to some day perform xenografts.

GVH PHENOMENON

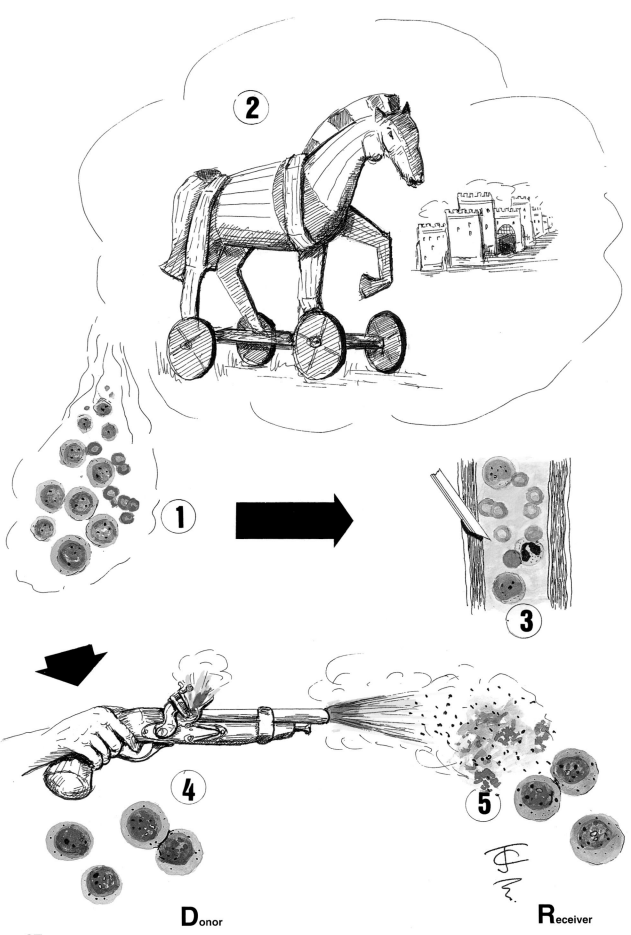

Donor

Receiver

Figure 67

3.6 Graft-Versus-Host Reaction (GVH)

In this type of reaction, it could be said that it is the graft which rejects the host. Immunologically competent T lymphocytes contained in the graft (mainly in bone marrow grafts) attack cells of the receiver, and in acute forms may provoke immunologically severe and even fatal lesions, involving liver, skin, and intestine. Grafts containing aggressive lymphocytes are true Trojan horses introduced into the receiver's circulation, particularly when the receiver suffers from immune deficiency.

Figure 67 shows the GVH phenomenon: a bone marrow graft ❶ is introduced into the organism of the receiver ❸ like a "real" Trojan horse ❷. Once within the organism, T lymphocytes of the graft ❹ attack and kill lymphocytes of the receiver ❺. Of course, GVH reaction does not occur in autologous bone marrow grafts, where grafted cells are identical to those of the receiver.

Interestingly, the more intense but controlled a GVH reaction has been, the fewer are relapses of leukemia after bone marrow transplantation. This phenomenon, called graft-versus-leukemia reaction (GVL), is now under study.

Another promising line of research is the use of a **growth factor** in bone marrow grafts. This factor stimulates growth of stem cells, thus increasing the rate at which the graft takes.

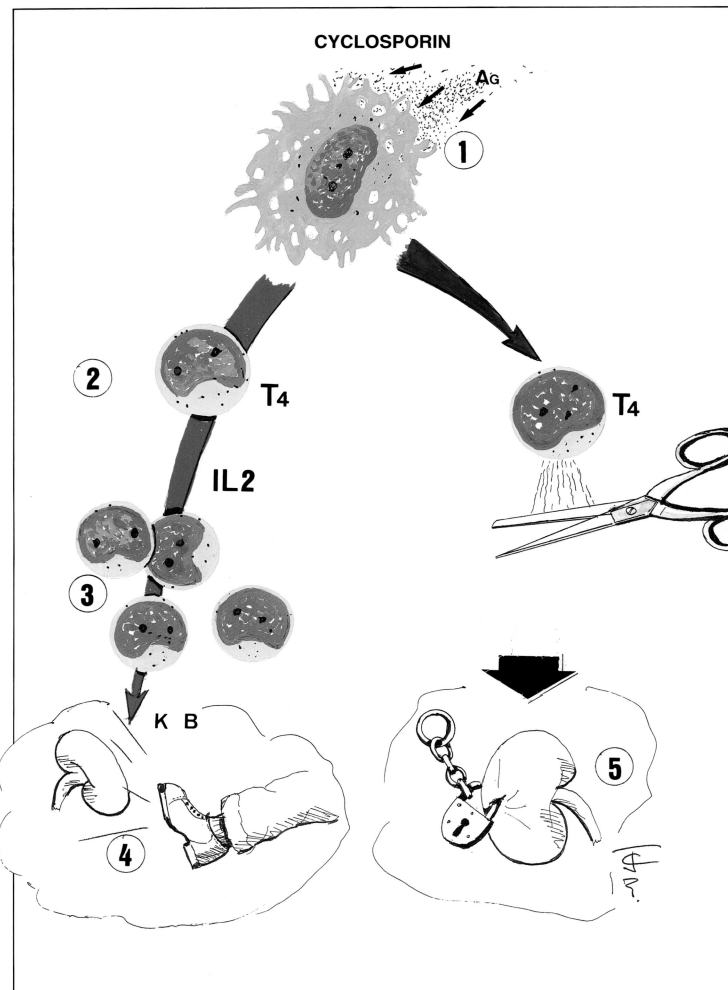

Figure 68

3.7 Immunosuppressive Therapies

The main indications for immunosuppressive therapy are organ transplantation and autoimmune diseases. The first immunosuppressive drugs were, on the one hand, antimitotic, i.e., acting on dividing cells, such as azathioprine, 6-mercaptopurine or methotrexate, and, on the other hand, corticosteroids, which suppress production of several lymphokines required for an immune response.

The discovery of cyclosporin has represented a major advance and has been followed by new derivatives with similar action, and also by other biological strategies based on anti-lymphocyte antibodies, immunotoxins or suppressor cytokines (e.g., IL-10).

Cyclosporin is an immunosuppressive extract of a mould (Tolypocladium). It has little general toxicity and is not cytostatic. It inhibits mainly the release of interleukin 2 and other lymphokines by T lymphocytes. As a result, there is a considerable reduction in proliferation of T4 lymphocytes and B lymphocytes. It may be recalled that interleukin 2 is synthesized by helper lymphocytes (T4) of the Th0 and Th1 classes, when they are stimulated by a macrophage.

Figure 68 shows the mechanism of action of cyclosporin.

❶ Macrophage phagocytizing antigens and presenting them to T4 lymphocytes.

❷ T4 lymphocytes secreting IL-2. This mediator stimulates proliferation of B lymphocytes and cytotoxic K lymphocytes (killer cells) ❸.

Cyclosporin is currently the main drug used in organ transplantation because it prevents rejection, which is provoked above all by cytotoxic T lymphocytes (K) and B lymphocytes ❹.

By neutralizing these lymphocytes, cyclosporin permits the graft to "take" ❺.

But, as always in immunotherapy, there are two sides to the coin. Suppression of K and B lymphocytes proliferation creates a risk of infection (particularly viral infections) and the appearance of lymphomas. Thus, careful dosage and therapeutic combinations must be observed.

Recently, indications of cyclosporin and other similar drugs acting on lymphokine production have been extended to other areas, such as autoimmune diseases including insulin-dependent diabetes, inflammatory diseases, such as cortico-resistent asthma and proliferative disorders, such as psoriasis.

Under some conditions, plasma exchange (plasmapheresis) or gammaglobulin injections may also have immunodepressive effects. The careful administration of immunosuppressive therapies is a delicate business, and is best left to specialists in this field.

AUTOIMMUNE DISEASES

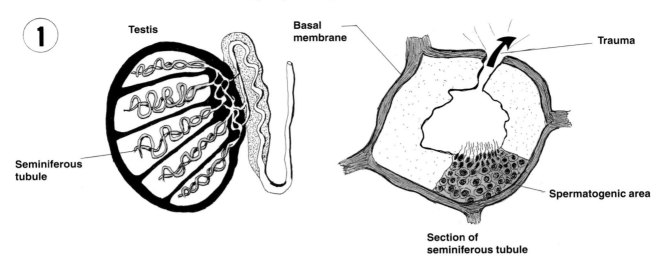

1

Testis

Basal membrane

Trauma

Seminiferous tubule

Spermatogenic area

Section of seminiferous tubule

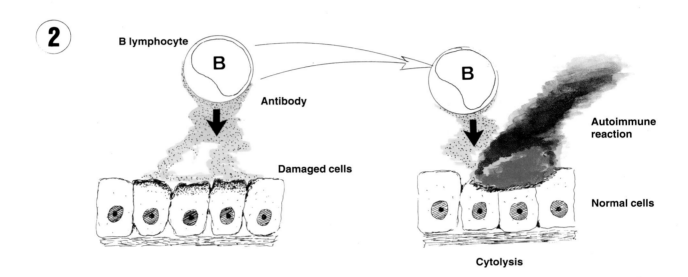

2

B lymphocyte

B

Antibody

Damaged cells

B

Autoimmune reaction

Normal cells

Cytolysis

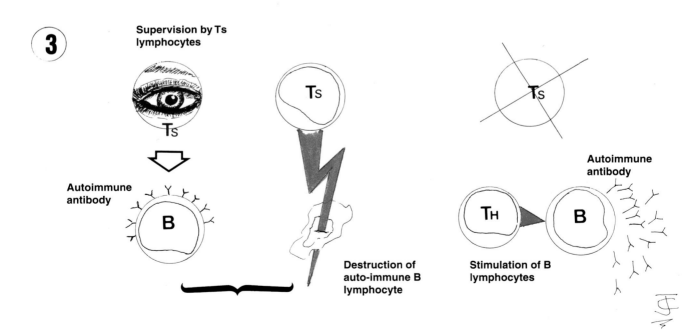

3

Supervision by Ts lymphocytes

T$_S$

T$_S$

Autoimmune antibody

B

Destruction of auto-immune B lymphocyte

Autoimmune antibody

T$_H$

B

Stimulation of B lymphocytes

Figure 69

3.8. Autoimmune Diseases

An organism does not, normally, react against its own constituents, since it recognizes them as "self." However, under abnormal conditions this equilibrium may be upset and the organism may manufacture humoral antibodies and immunocompetent lymphoid cells directed against its own tissue antigens. It is important to distinguish between **autoimmune reactions and autoimmune diseases**. An **autoimmune reaction** has no known pathological consequences. It may be no more than a control reaction or, even more probably, a reaction aimed at removing degraded substances which become autoantigenic. Thus, after myocardial infarction, anti-cardiac antibodies are found in serum. This type of antibody is not known to have pathological effects.

In **autoimmune diseases**, on the other hand, the immune response does have certain pathological consequences. The mechanism of these autoimmune reactions is not clearly understood at present. Several hypotheses have been put forward, but none is entirely satisfactory.

Hypothesis 1: Sequestered antigens (Figure 69) ❶. There appear to be antigens in spermatozoa and in the crystalline lens of the eye which have no contact with the immune system. Thus, in the case of the testicles, the seminiferous tubules are completely isolated from the immune system. If some inflammatory disease or trauma occurs, cells up to that time unknown to the immune system may emerge and come into contact with the body's lymphocytes. A well-known example is **orchitis**, a complication of mumps. Similarly, **"sympathetic ophthalmia"** appears following trauma to one eye, causing immunological lesions spreading to the other eye. Cells which up to now have never been in contact with the individual's defense system are considered to be foreign and are not recognized, hence the harmful immune response.

Hypothesis 2: Modified antigens. Normally, the body recognizes its own cells, but if cells have been modified by a drug, radiation, chemicals, or an infectious agent, they may become different and no longer recognizable as self. **Figure 69 ❷** shows, on the left, damaged cells and a B lymphocyte manufacturing antibodies against these cells. The same series of sensitized B lymphocytes is shown on the right, directing their antibodies against normal cells of the organism and causing cytolysis. Only minimal modification of autologous cells is sufficient to be no longer recognized as self. The immune response towards modified cells damages normal cells by immune cross-reaction. The classical example of this phenomenon is the appearance of hemolytic antistreptococcal antibodies attacking not only streptococci but also heart valve tissues. Streptococci and heart tissue are thought to have common antigenic determinants. Consequently, endocarditis may develop. This theory is not unanimously accepted. It has been used as an argument against bacteriological vaccines, but has not yet been conclusively proven.

Hypothesis 3: This probably comes closest to the truth, but it is also the most difficult to prove. In **Figure 69 ❸** are shown, on the left Ts (suppressor) lymphocytes monitoring B lymphocytes. If abnormal antibodies appear on the surface of B lymphocytes, Ts cells destroy them immediately (elimination of **"forbidden clones"**).

In autoimmune diseases, Ts lymphocytes are supposed to become disoriented. At that moment, B lymphocytes, which are no longer monitored, manufacture antibodies which may be directed against cells of the organism. B cells are, moreover, also stimulated by Th (helper) cells.

Although the mechanisms of autoimmunity are not yet clearly understood, this phenomenon plays a major role in medicine. A few examples of autoimmune reactions and diseases include: encephalitis after vaccination against rabies, encephalitis after chickenpox or rubella vaccination, multiple sclerosis, sympathetic ophthalmia, orchitis after mumps, Hashimoto's thyroiditis, Biermer's anemia, systemic lupus erythematosus, rheumatoid arthritis, etc.

In many cases, antibodies responsible for or accompanying autoimmune reactions are directed against cellular nuclei (**antinuclear antibodies, ANA**).

These antibodies are directed against one or several of the multiple components of the cell nucleus, especially against DNA (deoxyribonucleic acid). In some diseases, mainly connective-tissue disorders or collagenoses, antibodies are found in the blood, capable of provoking severe immunological lesions. They are identified particularly by indirect immunofluorescence.

These antibodies are manifold and their identification, particularly from their appearance under the microscope when fixed to cells, permits the specialist to determine their nature. The main diseases in which antinuclear antibodies are found are: systemic lupus erythematosus, Sjögren's syndrome, scleroderma, polymyositis, rheumatoid arthritis, etc. It should be noted, however, that ANA are not entirely specific to these diseases.

ANTINUCLEAR ANTIBODIES (ANA)

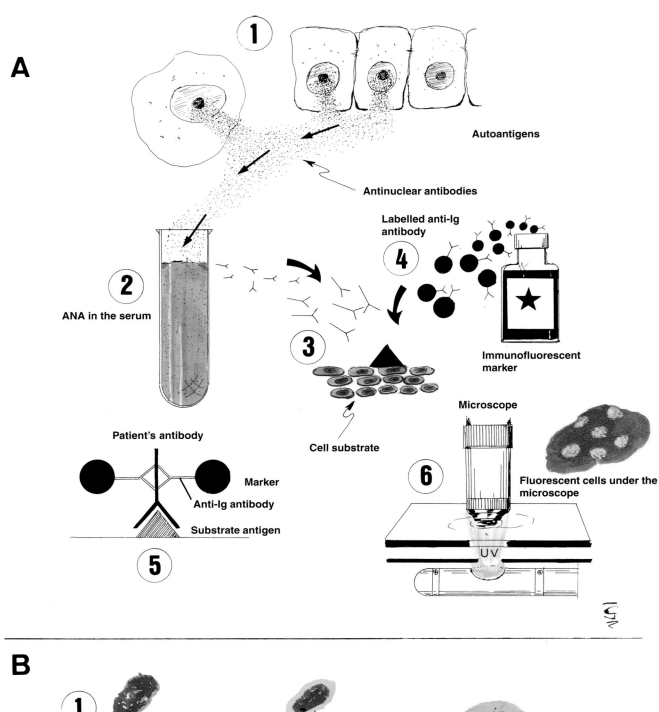

A

1

Autoantigens

Antinuclear antibodies

2

ANA in the serum

4

Labelled anti-Ig antibody

Immunofluorescent marker

3

Cell substrate

Patient's antibody

5

Marker

Anti-Ig antibody

Substrate antigen

Microscope

6

UV

Fluorescent cells under the microscope

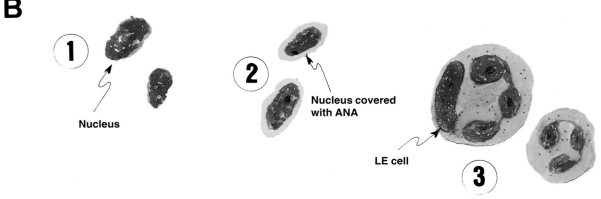

B

1

Nucleus

2

Nucleus covered with ANA

LE cell

3

Figure 70

Figure 70 A shows the demonstration of ANA by **immunofluorescence**. In ❶, antigens specific to nuclei are shown leaving the cell and inducing antibody formation by stimulation of the immune system. These antibodies are found in the patient's serum ❷. Indirect immunofluorescence technique is applied, using as substrate, i. e., as antigen, nucleated cells containing a maximum of proteins and nucleic acid ❸. Serum containing the antibodies is then put in contact with these cells. The black triangle in ❸ shows the antigen, consisting of such cells rich in nuclear elements (especially DNA). At present, cells used are mostly human larynx cancer cells, sections of rat kidney or liver or, more recently, a protozoan, Crithidia Lucilia, containing large amounts of DNA.

In ❹, a marker (colored anti-antibody), which becomes fluorescent under UV light, is added to the antigen-antibody complex (antigen being represented by cell nuclei as a substrate, and antibody being the patient's serum). In ❺ is represented the immunofluorescence reaction: substrate antigen + patient's serum antibody + fluorescent marker. In ❻, the preparation is exposed to UV light, which renders the fluorescent dye visible under the microscope. Fluorescent cells stand out against the dark background (yellow-green when fluorescein is used as a marker). Cells visible under the microscope are substrate cells, which retain the serum's ANAs. In this way, it can be ascertained that ANA are present in serum.

In **Figure 70 B**, ❶ shows nuclei of cells that have been targets of ANA (antinucleoprotein): the protoplasm has been destroyed. In ❷, these nuclei are covered with antinuclear antibodies, rendering them recognizable by intact polymorphonuclears. In ❸, the cell nucleus is phagocytosed by a polynuclear cell, producing a characteristic picture: next to the nucleus of the victim cell, the nucleus of the polynuclear may be seen. This is a **Hargraves' cell or "LE-cell,"** found in several diseases, such as systemic lupus erythematosus (SLE), particularly in bone marrow cells removed by sternal puncture.

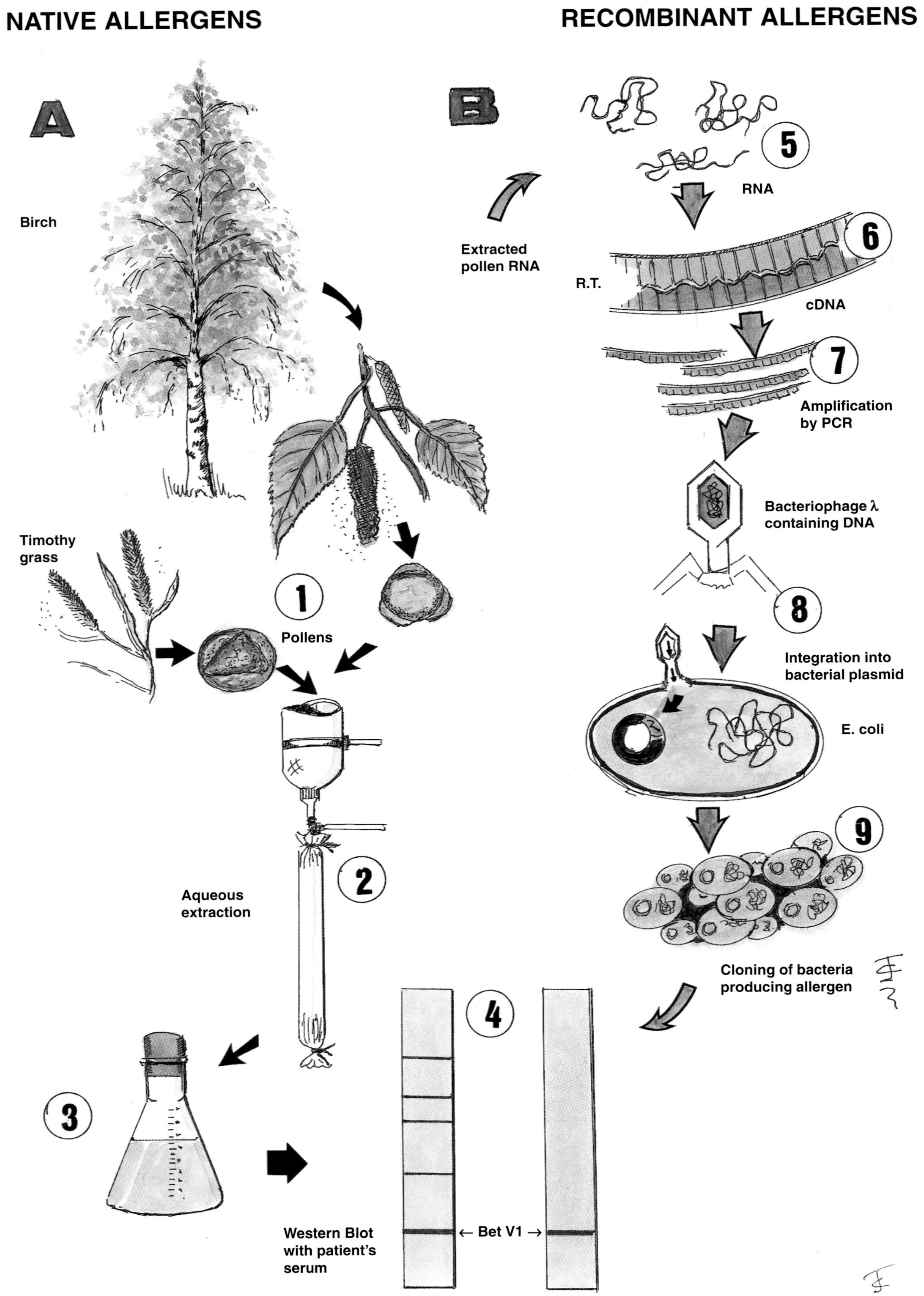

NATIVE ALLERGENS

RECOMBINANT ALLERGENS

A

Birch

Timothy grass

1 Pollens

2 Aqueous extraction

3

4 Western Blot with patient's serum ← Bet V1 →

B

5 RNA

Extracted pollen RNA

6 R.T. cDNA

7 Amplification by PCR

Bacteriophage λ containing DNA

8 Integration into bacterial plasmid

E. coli

9 Cloning of bacteria producing allergen

Figure 71

Part Four

Allergens and Vaccines

4.1 Native and Recombinant Allergens

Allergens used in allergy diagnosis, e. g., in skin tests or in specific immunotherapy, are generally obtained by aqueous extraction **(Figure 71 ❷)** from raw materials such as pollens, foods, animal danders, insect venoms, moulds, house dust mite cultures etc., as shown in **Figure 71, ❶**. Such allergens are qualified as native: the components acting as allergens are mostly proteins but some allergens are polysaccharides.

Such an extraction procedure is very empirical: numerous substances beside the desired allergens are simultaneously extracted and the quality of an allergen extract is highly dependent upon the purity and homogeneity of the raw materials used for extraction. Quantitative determination of allergens present in a given extract and their standardization are still posing numerous problems. At the onset, allergen content was expressed as **weight/volume (Noon units),** based on the weight of raw material in relation to the fluid volume used for extraction. Obviously, reproducibility of such a procedure may only be very approximate. Later, the **amount of protein nitrogen (PNU)** present in the final extract was determined. This procedure is likewise not satisfactory, because numerous non-allergenic proteins may contaminate the final extract, as suggested in **Figure 71, ❹**.

Nowadays, allergen standardization involves serological methods (e. g., reaction with specific IgE determined by inhibition of a standardized RAST test, or skin tests with various allergen dilutions in a group of allergic patients. These procedures lead to the definition of **biological units** (e. g., the **AU Unit,** defined by a standardized skin test procedure from the American FDA, or the **HEP Unit,** defined by a Scandinavian procedure). Unfortunately, there is not yet a universally recognized international biological unit. Concerted efforts by research scientists, pharmaceutical industries and control authorities have already yielded considerable improvements in recent years in the quality of allergenic extracts for the major allergens used in diagnosis and specific therapy.

These efforts likewise permitted isolation and identification of a certain number of molecules in allergenic extracts representing **major allergens.** A major allergen (e. g., Bet

V1 protein in birch pollen extract) may be identified as such because the majority of the immune response of allergic individuals, particularly specific IgE antibodies, is directed against such a molecule, or because most people allergic and reacting to the whole allergen extract are sensitized to that major allergen. Isolation and purification of protein allergens permitted definition of their structures and of the structure of the corresponding DNA.

This advance led through classical procedures of molecular biology to entire in vitro synthesis of **recombinant allergens.** The big advantage of recombinant allergens is that their homogeneous structure **(Figure 71)** is entirely known and their preparation eminently reproducible. The various steps encompass extraction of pollen RNA **(Figure 71 ❺)**, transcription into DNA ❻ and its multiplication by PCR ❼, followed by expression of DNA in a bacteriophage ❽, integration into an E. coli plasmid and cloning of bacteria ❾. This technology likewise permits us to produce rare allergens in unlimited amounts, particularly when procurement of raw materials is difficult. In principle, recombinant allergens should enable us to markedly improve the quality of allergy diagnosis and immunotherapy. Nonetheless, one problem remains: most raw materials and allergen extracts against which our patients are sensitized contain more than a single major allergen, indeed several very different allergenic molecules. Accordingly, complete reconstitution by molecular biology of the vast range of native allergens is a far reaching enterprise of doubtful economic interest. In addition, this approach is probably only valid for allergens of exclusively proteinic nature.

Nevertheless, the arrival of recombinant allergens, the list of which is already long, provides for the first time well defined molecules as allergens in allergological research. Likewise, we may now envisage new approaches to the specific treatment of allergies, e. g., in form of allergen fragments inducing immunological tolerance (T cell epitopes) or in form of mixed vaccines, where the DNA portion of the allergen is linked to an inoffensive retrovirus, enabling permanent contact with allergen in the allergic patient, to whom such a vaccine would be administered (see as an analogy 4.5, vaccination of fish with similar mixed vaccines)

NEUTRALIZATION OF TOXINS

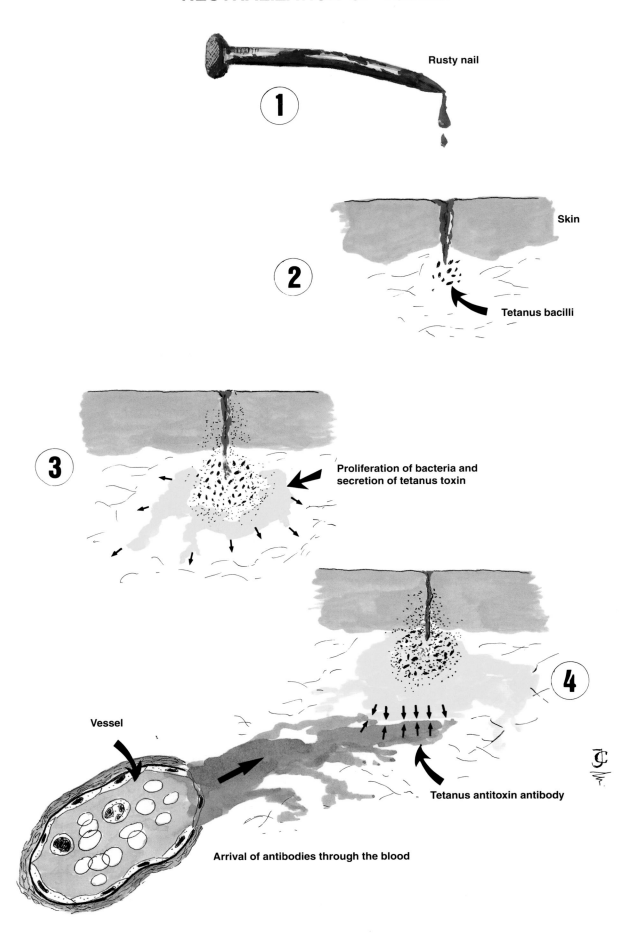

Rusty nail

1

Skin

2

Tetanus bacilli

3

Proliferation of bacteria and secretion of tetanus toxin

4

Vessel

Tetanus antitoxin antibody

Arrival of antibodies through the blood

Figure 72

4.2 Antitoxin, Antimicrobial, and Antiviral Vaccines

Antibodies are able to neutralize microbial toxins, provided they are present in sufficient quantities. This applies to tetanus, diphtheria, botulism, gangrene, etc. These antibodies are present in the organism only following an initial immunogenic infection. The primary reaction causes the appearance of specific antibodies secreted by plasmocytes and the awakening of B memory cells. It is B memory cells which, during renewed infection, are transformed in plasmocytes which very quickly synthesize specific antibodies. Vaccination against bacteria or viruses (e. g., poliomyelitis) creates this **immunological memory.** Vaccination is carried out with killed bacteria or attenuated viruses, i.e those which have been slightly modified compared to original bacteria or viruses. Antibodies synthesized in this way closely resemble antibodies induced by living bacteria or viruses. There is **cross antigenicity**. In some diseases, in which the infectious element is a **toxin**, vaccination is carried out with chemically neutralized toxins, called **anatoxins or toxoids**. The principle is the same: the anatoxin is antigenically similar to the toxin, but does not possess its toxic effects.

Figure 72 shows what happens in the case of tetanus infection. ❶ The proverbial rusty nail, carrying tetanus bacteria. In ❷, the wound caused by the nail is neither deep nor serious, but it is enough to permit development of anaerobic tetanus bacteria, i. e., bacteria not needing oxygen for their multiplication. The small microbial colony quickly secretes highly virulent toxins ❸. Antibodies present in the blood immediately rush to neutralize the toxins ❹. If the individual does not carry any antibodies, either because he has not been vaccinated or because he has never been infected before, he has to be injected with prepared antibodies, as he will not have enough time to synthesize his own. This is known as **serotherapy**, i. e., the injection of serum containing specific antibodies. To avoid reactions to horse immunoglobulins (horses have long been used as source for therapeutic serum), antisera based on specific human γ-globulins are increasingly used.

Vaccination is therefore the use of antigenic substances to force the organism to manufacture its own antibodies, whereas **serotherapy** is the use of prepared antibodies ready to act in cases where there is no time for vaccination.

The use of recombinant bacterial or viral antigens or even of synthetic antigens has recently allowed great progress in the field of vaccines.

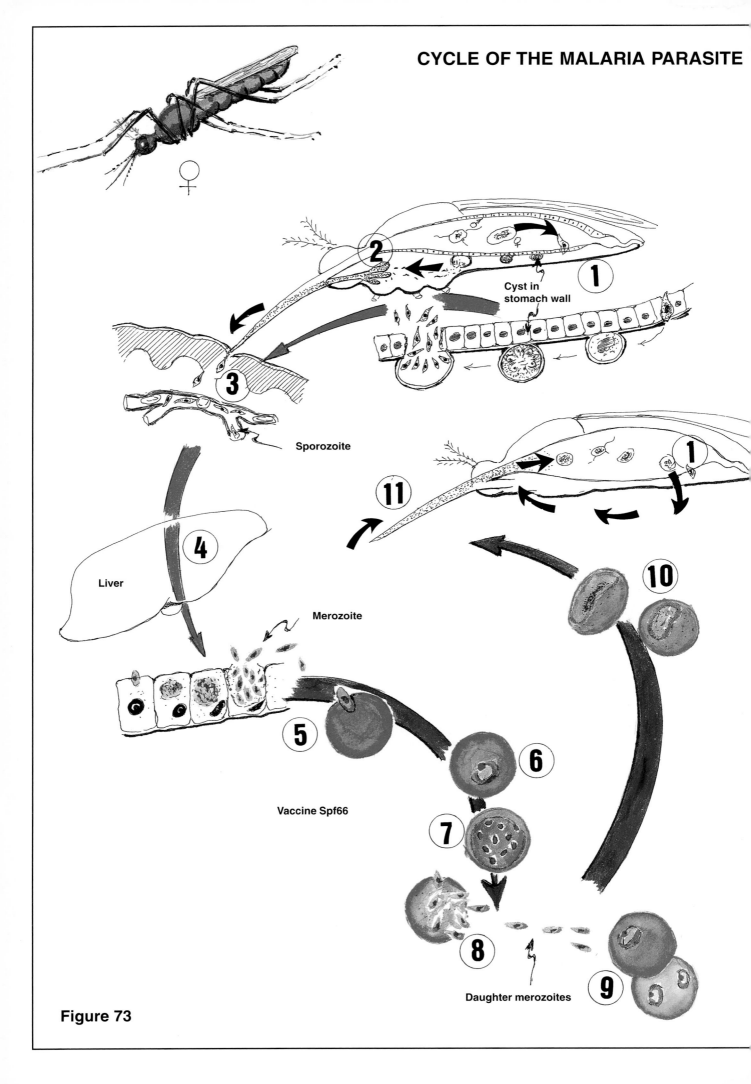

CYCLE OF THE MALARIA PARASITE

Cyst in stomach wall

Sporozoite

Liver

Merozoite

Vaccine Spf66

Daughter merozoites

Figure 73

4.3 Malaria: the Search for a Vaccine. The Difficulties

Malaria is one of the most widespread diseases in the world: it is responsible for 300–400 million cases in tropical countries, and one to three million deaths annually in tropical Africa, particularly among children less than 5 years of age. It is the main cause of severe anemia and of many, often fatal, complications .

Chronic malaria often creates partial immunity, appearing often only after the age of six, an immunity maintained by continual reinfections. Travelers who fail to take strict protective measures are at great risk, since a single mosquito bite may be lethal. The same applies to Africans and Asians returning home after staying for one or two years in a temperate zone.

Furthermore, strains of mosquitoes (anopheles) resistant to insecticides are appearing, as are malaria parasites resistant to conventional antimalaria drugs (quinine, chloroquine, etc.) This is especially the case for Plasmodium falciparum, considered to be the most pathogenic. Numerous drugs have been tested: they are often effective but toxic. Hence our interest in developing a vaccine.

4.3.1 The parasite cycle

To understand the complexity of the problem, let us recall the cycle of the parasite **(Figure 73)**.

A female Anopheles mosquito infects man with the parasite at the stage of **sporozoites** ❸. These move quickly within the bloodstream to the liver ❹. It is during this short period (20–30 minutes) that the parasites are thought to be vulnerable to antibodies. Unfortunately, they are later protected inside the liver cells ❺, where they multiply, each sporozoite producing 2000–40,000 **merozoites** (within 6 weeks at most). These merozoites enter the red blood cells ❺ ❻ by means of a membrane receptor. There, they are again protected from antibodies and immune lymphocytes. They multiply ❼, each merozoite producing 6–24 daughter merozoites ❽. Each parasite is capable of reinfecting a red blood cell ❾ and provoking hemolysis, with clinical attacks of malaria.

Up to this point, multiplication is asexual. Sexual forms then appear: male and female **gametocytes** ❿. These are present in the small skin vessels and are aspirated by the mosquito ⓫⓬. Gametocytes are fertilized in the mosquito's stomach ❶ to form a cyst in its stomach wall. Finally, numerous sporozoites form in these cysts and migrate to the mosquito's salivary glands ❷. The cycle starts then all over again.

4.3.2 Attempts to produce a malaria vaccine

The complexity of the Plasmodium cycle indicates the extreme difficulty encountered in producing a vaccine. The antigens vary throughout the cycle. In addition, the many varieties of plasmodia do not help to solve the problem. Currently the most valid approach is vaccination against sporozoites, e. g., with sporozoites attenuated by X-ray exposure. If a single parasite escapes, vaccination fails. Nonetheless, such a vaccine could partially protect the traveler.

Thanks to MAbs, membrane receptors have been identified which enable merozoites to fix onto and penetrate red blood cells. Attempts have also been made to elicit antibodies against gametocytes. A vaccine against gametocytes would protect the community but not the individual. Since parasites inside liver cells and red blood cells are protected from antibodies and lymphocytes, attempts to target "armed" MAbs are being carried out, i. e., by using antibodies transporting antimalarial drugs (primaquine) towards liver cells.

The production of polyvalent vaccines acting at various stages of the parasite cycle could be a solution, but at what price?

Among the many problems inherent in the production of vaccines was the requirement to culture the parasite, but this has been achieved. The next step is to identify, within the Plasmodium, the genes responsible for synthesis of antigenic proteins; finally, we need sufficient quantities of the antigen.

Thanks to genetic engineering, specific genes of the parasite (recombinant DNA of Plasmodium falciparum) have been introduced into Escherichia coli as vector and permitted to produce large quantities of specific antigen.

Vaccination studies have shown that resistant individuals are those who have a high titter of antibodies against the sporozoite antigens. As a first step, investigators should develop a vaccine against sporozoites. Development of the parasite in the liver would also be blocked by the defenses provided by T lymphocytes, and perhaps by production of interferon. Briefly, to cover the various stages would require us to produce antibodies against sporozoites, preventing invasion of liver and red blood cells. We must then produce antibodies against merozoites, preventing multiplication in the blood and internal organs, and as a consequence reducing mortality and transmission.

Finally, production of antibodies against the gametes would prevent transmission to the community. The final result of vaccination should, in theory, be a mixture of antibodies directed against the various antigens appearing during the parasite cycle.

The most advanced vaccine currently in human trials (SPf66) is a synthetic vaccine made from various peptides of Plasmodium falciparum. It exerts its action during the red blood cell phase of the cycle, as illustrated in **Figure 73, ❺**.

In this entire area, there are many major unsolved problems, and intensive research is going on. Currently, several types of vaccines are in development. Of course similar problems occur in the development of AIDS vaccines.

Even if such vaccines could be developed, vaccination of entire populations would present another set of challenging social and economic problems.

Other solutions than vaccines are also being studied, involving biogenetic and ecologic approaches.

BIOLOGICAL INSECTICIDE

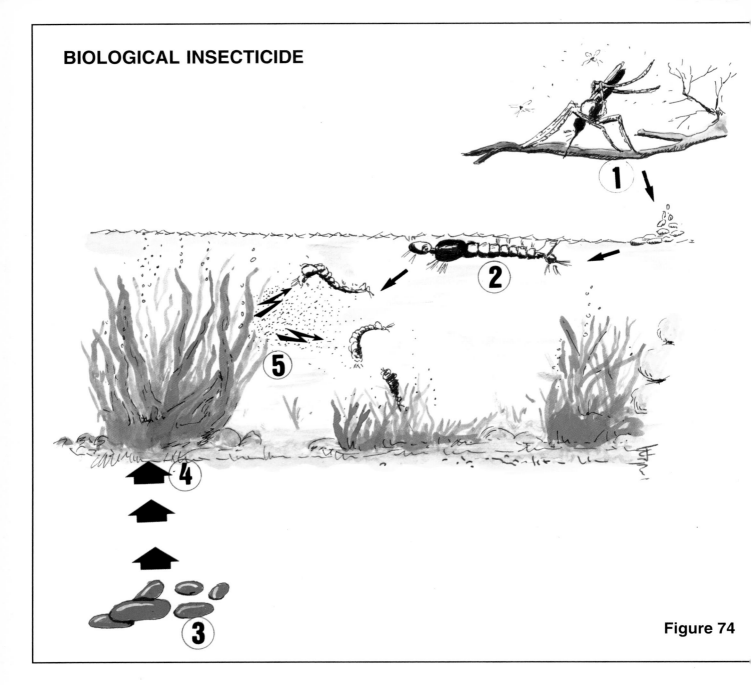

Figure 74

4.3.3 Genetic engineering to the rescue of immunology

The fight against malaria has also included, in a first stage, elimination of the vector mosquitoes by insecticides. Insecticides, however, are double-edged weapons, owing to their pollutant and toxic action (e. g., the indestructible DDT) as well as to their ability of inducing resistant strains of mosquitoes.

In contrast, "biological" insecticides do not pollute. Among numerous approaches, biotechnology has made possible isolation and culture of a microorganism called *Bacillus thuringiensis*, an insecticidal bacterium.

The genes of this microorganism, coding for a specific toxic protein with insecticide effect, have been isolated and injected into blue-green algae, which are present universally in freshwater where mosquito larvae develop, among them those carrying malaria (Anopheles), yellow fever, and onchocerciasis.

As a result, these algae produce a protein toxic for mosquito larvae. The idea to use a "bioinsecticide" based on microorganisms is already relatively old. This procedure has been used industrially in order to produce insecticide powders. The masterstroke lies in letting the insecticide be produced directly by genetic manipulation of the algae, which is a required food for the mosquitoes. Further very interesting studies are under way.

We have taken this brief digression into biotechnology to show that, although vaccination against malaria has come up against very difficult obstacles, other approaches to fighting this disease are being carefully considered. The least we can say is that some of these approaches are quite imaginative.

Figure 74 shows in ❶ a mosquito laying its eggs on water. In ❷, the mosquito larvae. In ❸, Bacillus thuringiensis, the genes of which have been inserted into blue-green algae ❹. The toxin secreted by these algae kill mosquito larvae ❺.

4.4 Research and Hopes in Immune Therapy of Cancer

For a long time, physicians have sought to treat cancer by immune therapy. Since the immune system destroys cells attacked by viruses or microbes, neutralizes toxins, and rejects transplants recognized as foreign, why should it not also reject cells which have been modified by cancer?

Burnet's theory suggests that since our defense system rejects systematically all abnormal cells the appearance of cancer must imply the failure of our surveillance system. This theory has not been confirmed.

Here the main conclusions of multiple studies devoted to the immunology of cancers are briefly summarized.

1) Tumors **experimentally induced** in mice by chemical carcinogens may express immunogenic tumoral antigens leading to cancer rejection.
2) **Spontaneous** murine tumors may carry specific tumoral antigens which, however, **are either weakly or not at all immunogenic,** and do not induce tumor rejection **(Figure 75)**.
3) The discovery of **monoclonal antibodies (MAb)** brought about an immunological revolution, but it was soon realized that they do not suffice to induce tumor rejection. The ephemeral dream of the "magic bullet" has been discussed earlier.
4) Recently, it has been shown **(Figure 76 A)** that non-immunogenic murine tumor cells, when treated with a mutagenic agent, lose their capacity to induce a pregredient tumor because they express **new antigens** able to induce **efficient rejection** similar to graft rejection. This is due to **cytotoxic T lymphocytes (LyTc).**
5) Attempts to isolate antigens responsible for tumor rejection have usually failed. However, some genes coding for antigens recognized by cytotoxic T lymphocytes have been identified (in cases of melanoma, a gene called MAGE1)
6) LyTc only recognize antigenic peptides when coupled to a MHC molecule **(Figure 21)**. In melanoma, the gene MAGE1 codes for an antigenic peptide forming within the cytoplasm of the tumor cell and ultimately localizing in a cleft of the HLA-A1 molecule. This complex **MAGE peptide + HLA-1** (called AgE) migrates towards the surface of the tumor cell and forms there the **cancer antigen responsible for rejection (Figure 76 B).**

This complex is recognized by LyTc. In view of the fact that not all antigenic peptides may bind to the HLA-A1 molecule and that, on the other hand, not all patients possess this HLA-A1 histocompatibility antigen, the number of candidates capable of rejecting their tumor by this particular MAGE peptide and mechanism is unfortunately quite limited (i. e., about 10% of human melanomas).

7) Several other cells or molecules may intervene in tumor rejection. NK cells, macrophages, and certain cytokines (TNF, IFN, IL-2) activating cells involved in rejection should be mentioned here.

Based on concepts summarized above, several strategies for immune therapy of cancers have been devised. But in view to the numerous still open questions, will they be efficacious?

Some of the approaches to **immune therapy of cancer** can be quickly summarized here:

1) Injecting the patient with tumor cells which have been killed, e. g., by X irradiation, and which are carrying a rejection antigen (e. g., in melanoma, MAGE1 peptide + HLA-A1), in order to activate Tc lymphocytes **(Figure 77)**. In such cells, one could also introduce the gene coding for IL-2 in order to amplify the response of lymphocytes present in their vicinity.
2) Insertion of a tumoral gene, such as MAGE1, in the DNA of a harmless virus and penetration of that virus in human cells, which would then express the antigenic tumoral peptide. This, combined with HLA antigens of those cells could induce an efficient lymphocyte reaction **(Figure 78)**.

IMMUNOTHERAPY OF CANCER

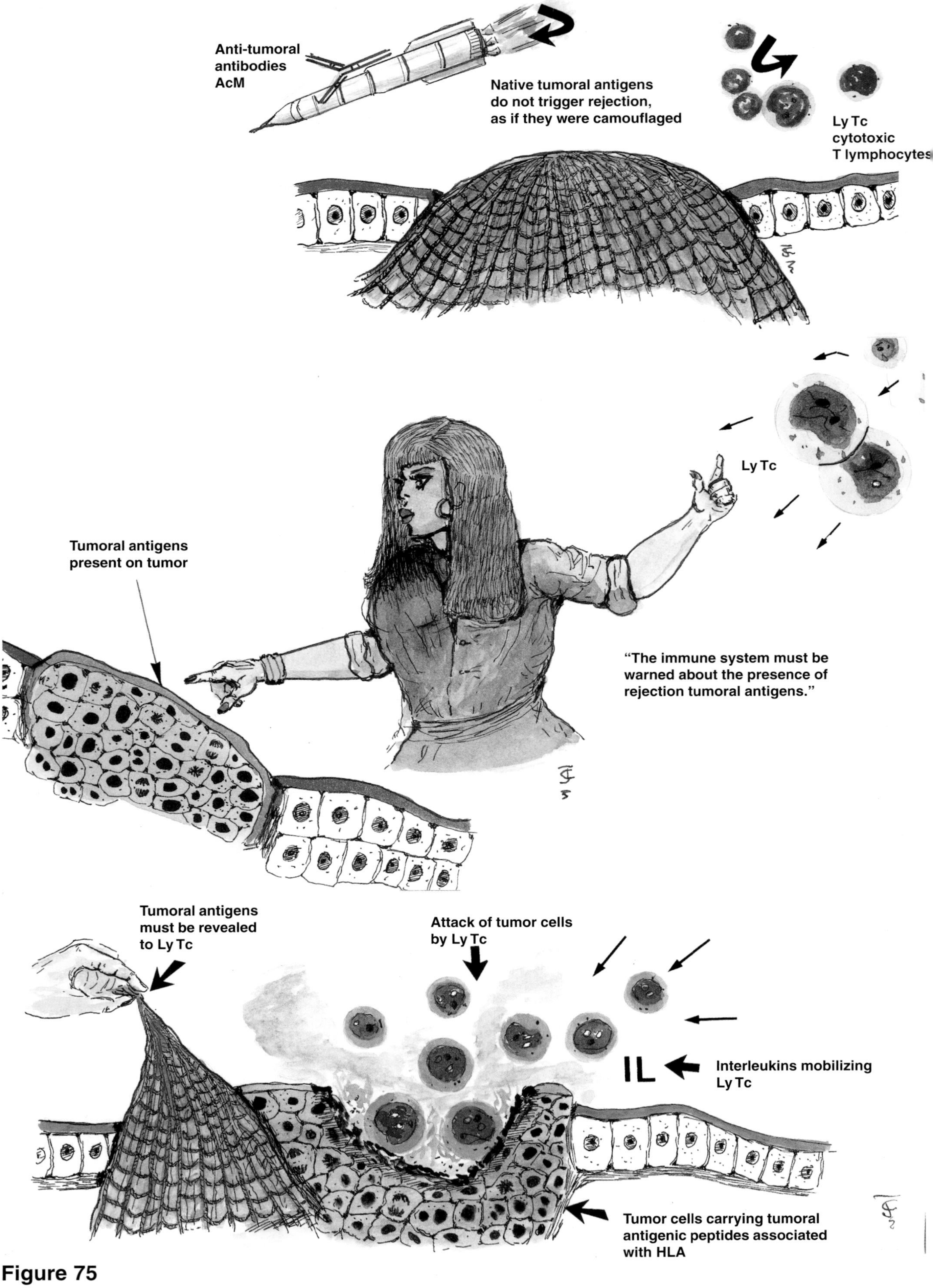

Anti-tumoral antibodies AcM

Native tumoral antigens do not trigger rejection, as if they were camouflaged

Ly Tc cytotoxic T lymphocytes

Ly Tc

Tumoral antigens present on tumor

"The immune system must be warned about the presence of rejection tumoral antigens."

Tumoral antigens must be revealed to Ly Tc

Attack of tumor cells by Ly Tc

Interleukins mobilizing Ly Tc

IL

Tumor cells carrying tumoral antigenic peptides associated with HLA

Figure 75

INDUCTION OF AN ANTI-TUMORAL IMMUNE RESPONSE

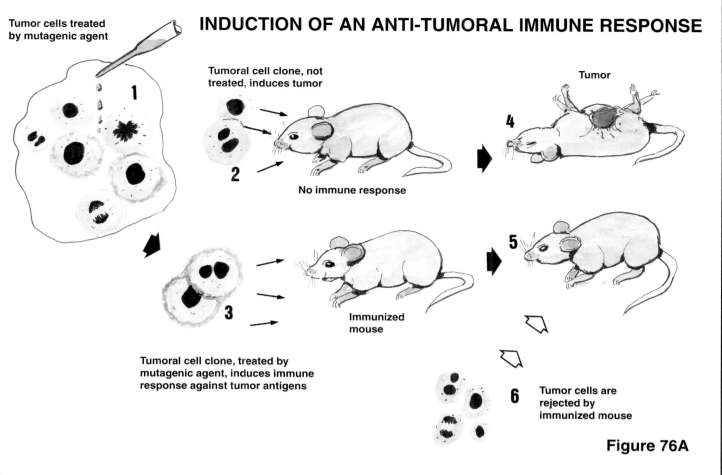

Tumor cells treated by mutagenic agent

1

Tumoral cell clone, not treated, induces tumor

2

No immune response

Tumor

4

Tumoral cell clone, treated by mutagenic agent, induces immune response against tumor antigens

3

Immunized mouse

5

6 Tumor cells are rejected by immunized mouse

Figure 76A

FORMATION OF TUMOR ANTIGENS AND RECOGNITION BY T LYMPHOCYTES

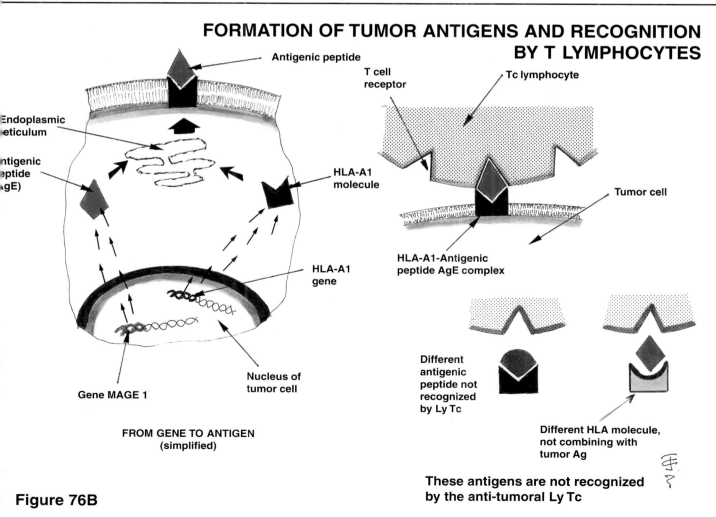

Antigenic peptide

Endoplasmic reticulum

Antigenic peptide (AgE)

HLA-A1 molecule

HLA-A1 gene

Nucleus of tumor cell

Gene MAGE 1

FROM GENE TO ANTIGEN (simplified)

T cell receptor

Tc lymphocyte

Tumor cell

HLA-A1-Antigenic peptide AgE complex

Different antigenic peptide not recognized by Ly Tc

Different HLA molecule, not combining with tumor Ag

These antigens are not recognized by the anti-tumoral Ly Tc

Figure 76B

NEW ATTEMPTS IN CANCER IMMUNOTHERAPY (1)

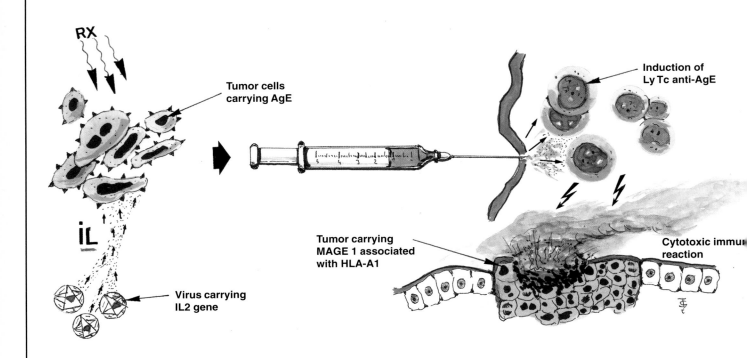

RX

Tumor cells carrying AgE

IL

Virus carrying IL2 gene

Induction of Ly Tc anti-AgE

Tumor carrying MAGE 1 associated with HLA-A1

Cytotoxic immun reaction

Figure 77

NEW ATTEMPTS IN CANCER IMMUNOTHERAPY (2)

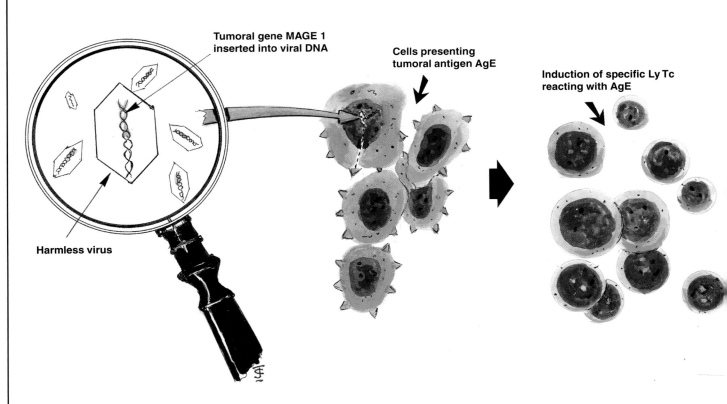

Tumoral gene MAGE 1 inserted into viral DNA

Cells presenting tumoral antigen AgE

Induction of specific Ly Tc reacting with AgE

Harmless virus

Figure 78

NEW ATTEMPTS IN CANCER IMMUNOTHERAPY (3 + 4)

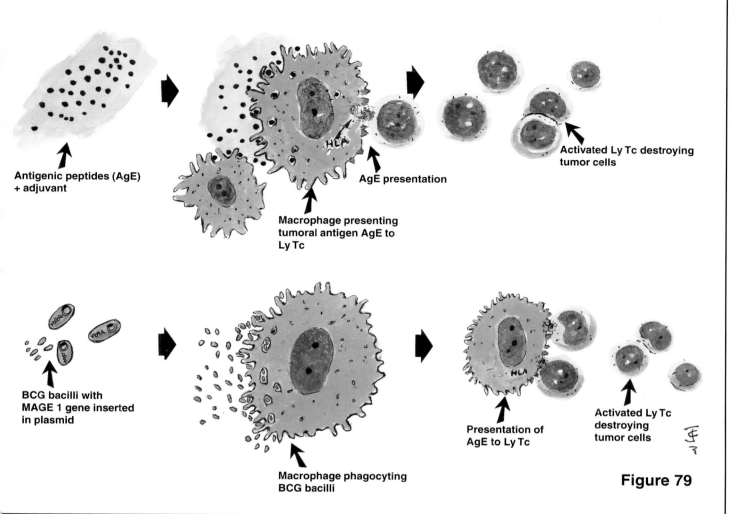

Antigenic peptides (AgE) + adjuvant

Macrophage presenting tumoral antigen AgE to Ly Tc

AgE presentation

Activated Ly Tc destroying tumor cells

BCG bacilli with MAGE 1 gene inserted in plasmid

Macrophage phagocyting BCG bacilli

Presentation of AgE to Ly Tc

Activated Ly Tc destroying tumor cells

Figure 79

3) Combination of an antigenic tumoral peptide (e.g., MAGE1) with an adjuvant. This mixture would be phagocyted by a macrophage carrying HLA-A1 and presented to Tc lymphocytes as tumor antigen inducing rejection. Then, activated lymphocytes would attack the tumor cells carrying MAGE1 and HLA-A1 **(Figure 79 ❸)**.

4) Recombination of a BCG (attenuated tuberculosis bacillus) plasmid with a tumoral gene, such as MAGE1. These modified bacteria would be phagocyted by macrophages

carrying HLA-A1, forming thereby a peptide-HLA complex. This would be presented to LyTc, inducing specific rejection of the tumor cells **(Figure 79, ❹)**.

Tumor genes other than MAGE1, the products of which combine with other HLA types and in other types of tumors, are currently being studied. The combination of several mechanisms acting simultaneously might be able to increase the efficacy of tumor "vaccines."

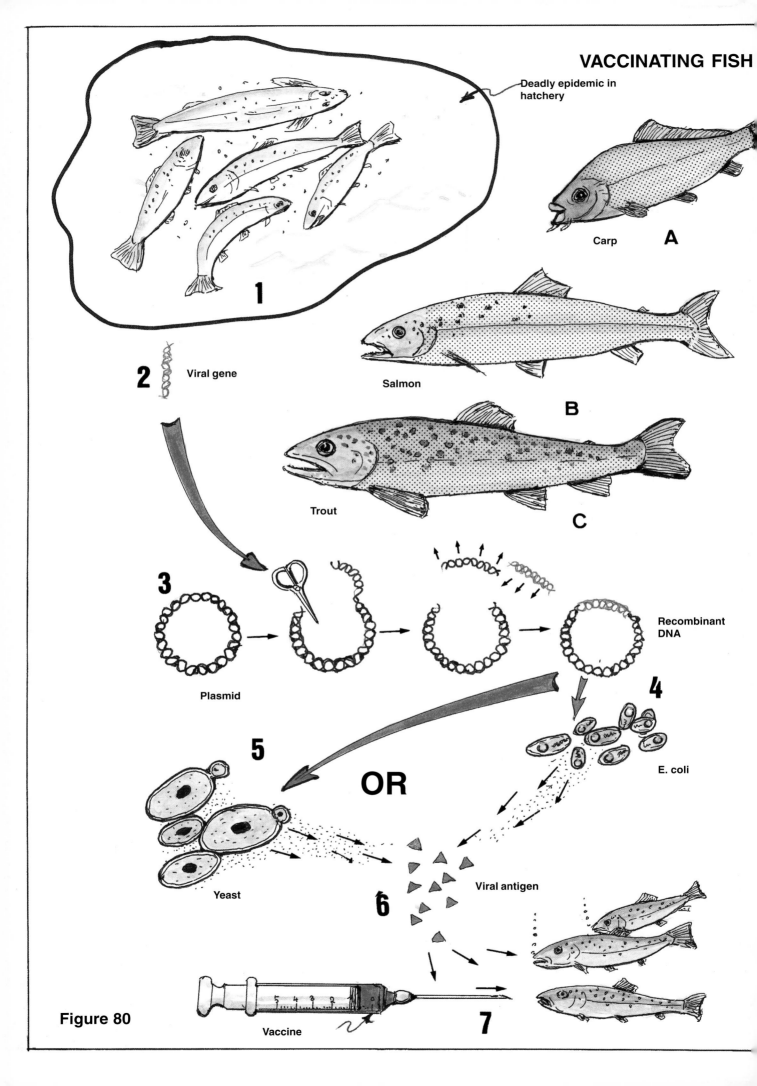

VACCINATING FISH

Deadly epidemic in hatchery

1

Carp **A**

Salmon **B**

Trout **C**

2 Viral gene

3 Plasmid

Recombinant DNA

4 E. coli

5 **OR**

Yeast

6 Viral antigen

7

Vaccine

Figure 80

4.5 Vaccination of Fish

Genetic engineering combined with immunology can sometimes open unexpected perspectives. Let us examine as an example the vaccination of fish.

In fish hatcheries, virus infections (rhabdovirus) may provoke severe damage and economic loss: one single infected fish may contaminate and destroy an entire pond.

In this context, the diseases of interest are mainly: spring viremia of carps **(Figure 80, A),** furonculosis and hematopoietic necrosis of salmon **(Figure 80, B),** and the hemorrhagic septicemia of trout **(Figure 80, C).** Thanks to sophisticated techniques using recombinant DNA, effective antiviral vaccines have been produced. A rough outline of this ingenious achievement is shown in **Figure 80**.

❶ Disaster following infection in a hatchery of carp (A), salmon (B) or trout (C).

❷ Specific viral gene extracted from virus cultures coming from infected fish. Nowadays, it is also possible to synthesize these genes, since their chemical structure is known.

❸ Gene cloned into a plasmid

❹ Plasmid introduced into Escherichia coli as vector

❺ or into yeast (Sachharomyces cerevisiae).

❻ These microorganism then produce viral antigens, which are either extracted, in the case of Escherichia coli, or directly secreted in the culture medium, in the case of yeast.

❼ Antigens are injected into the young fish ($\pm$ 15 g) thanks to an ingenious device. Vaccination is facilitated by letting fish swim in a partially anesthetic bath; oral administration of such vaccines is currently under study.

IMMUNODIFFUSION

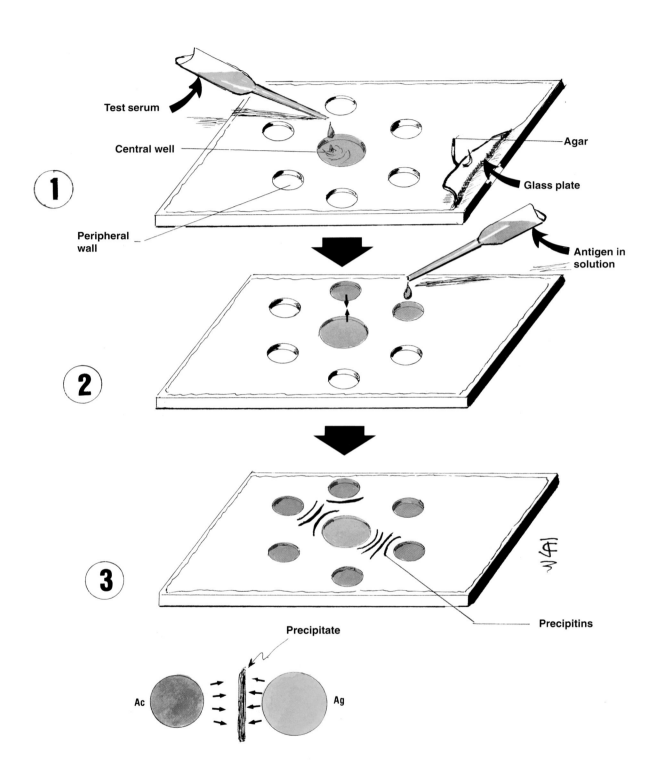

Figure 81

Part Five

Immunological Tests in vitro

Numerous immunological in-vitro tests, many with multiple variants, are currently available. We briefly discuss those which are the most widely used in diagnosis of allergic and immunological diseases.

5.1 Immunodiffusion

Immunodiffusion, developed by Ouchterlony, is one of the first methods that was used in clinical immunology **(Figure 81)**.

A layer of agar is poured onto a glass plate of similar size to that of a microscope slide. A central well with some peripheral wells are punched in the agar, and serum containing antibodies to be detected is poured in the central well ❶. Antigen solutions are poured into the peripheral wells ❷.

After some time, antigens diffuse in the agar towards antibody, and a precipitate appears in the region where the two substances meet. The precipitate ❸ is due to precipitating antibodies, which are of course called **precipitins.** Usually, these are immunoglobulins of the IgG or IgM class.

This technique is currently used to detect antibodies in a patient's blood against

– pigeon serum antigens (bird-fancier's lung),
– mouldy hay antigens (Farmer's lung),
– Aspergillus (causing transient pulmonary infiltrates), etc.

These diseases belong to type III allergy.

RADIAL IMMUNODIFFUSION ACCORDING TO MANCINI

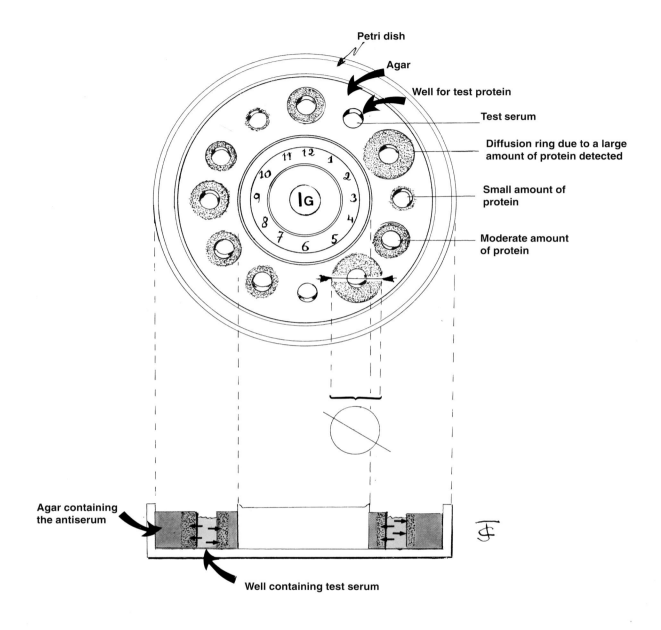

Figure 82

5.2 Determination of the Main Protein Fractions in Serum by Radial Immunodiffusion (Mancini's technique)

In practice, the most interesting immunological proteins in serum are: IgA, IgM, and IgG.

IgE and IgD are present in serum in amounts too low to be determined by simple immunodiffusion.

The technique of radial immunodiffusion, also called **Mancini's technique**, is remarkably easy to carry out **(Figure 82)**. Petri dishes containing agar with punched out wells are required. The sera to be tested are placed in the wells,

while an antibody specific for the serum antigen to be quantitatively evaluated is incorporated in the agar. A diffusion ring then appears around each well, with the ring diameter corresponding to the amount of antigen present in the well. This diameter is compared with a reference scale.

Special ready-for-use plates or dishes are available for each serum protein fraction to be tested, such as IgA, IgM, IgG, transferrin, antitrypsin, macroglobulin, etc.

ELECTROPHORESIS

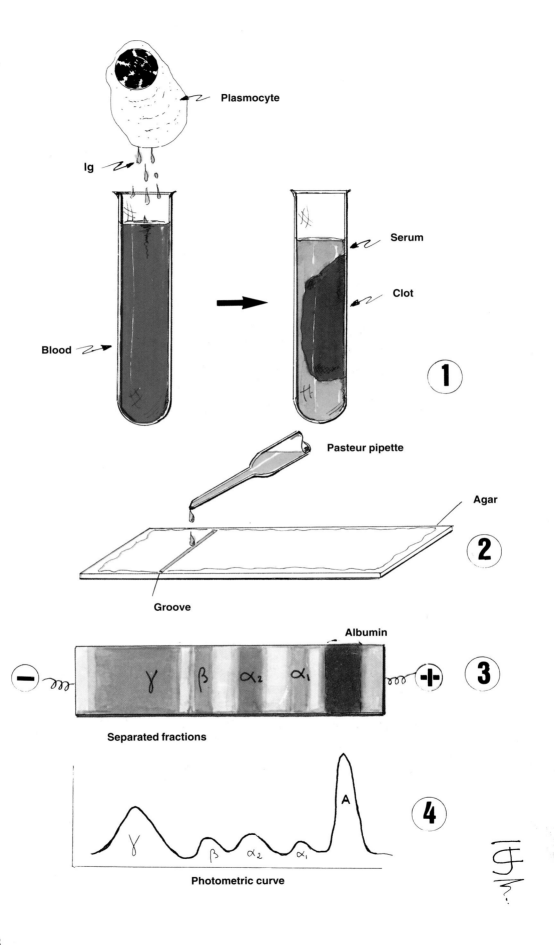

Plasmocyte

Ig

Blood

Serum

Clot

1

Pasteur pipette

Agar

Groove

2

Albumin

γ   β   α₂   α₁

Separated fractions

3

Photometric curve

4

Figure 83

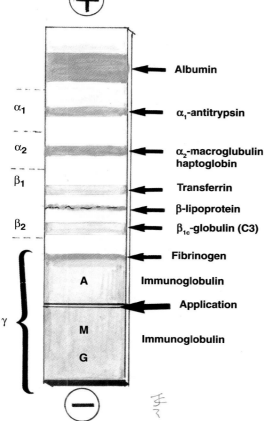

⊕

	← **Albumin**
α₁	← **α₁-antitrypsin**
α₂	← **α₂-macroglubulin haptoglobin**
β₁	← **Transferrin**
	← **β-lipoprotein**
β₂	← **β₁c-globulin (C3)**
	← **Fibrinogen**
γ { A	**Immunoglobulin**
	← **Application**
M G	**Immunoglobulin**

⊖

Figure 84

5.3 Protein Electrophoresis

In order to evaluate certain serum fractions, particularly γ-globulins, serum is first separated from the blood clot **(Figure 83)** ❶. Glass slides are covered with a layer of agar or gelose ❷, as for immunodiffusion.

A groove is punched at one end of the slide, perpendicular to its long axis. The serum to be tested is poured in this groove with a Pasteur pipette ❷. An electric current is then passed through the agar, which causes the various protein constituents of the serum to migrate in the agar medium. Each component migrates at its own pace, depending on its electric charge, on its molecular weight, on the density of the agar medium, etc., and other factors. When migration has been completed, the various components are separated and can be identified with a proper staining ❸.

The color density of each electrophoretic band is measured photometrically and a curve can be plotted ❹. The different bands of precipitation may also be simply examined with the naked eye.

In the electrophoresis shown here, it can be shown that albumin (A) migrates towards the positive pole, whereas the gammaglobulins, which interest us most, migrate towards the negative pole. The gammaglobulins form a mixture which gives a rather wide migration band.

The levels of the various fractions contained in serum are as follows, expressed in%:

– albumin: 50–60%
– α₁-globulins: 4–7%
– α₂-globulins: 5–9%
– β-globulins: 11–14%
– γ-globulins: 15–20%.

It is very important to interpret laboratory results correctly, as in most cases, normal values are given for adults. In newborns and infants, 16% of γ-globulins are found at birth, 4–5% after 2 months, and 8% after 1 year. This demonstrates the variations observed with age in infants.

Electrophoresis is a basic method, which underwent a number of improvements, especially much more detailed fractionations (e.g., migration in agarose **(Figure 84)** or polyacrylamide gel **(Figure 91)**, electrofocalization, etc.).

IMMUNOELECTROPHORESIS

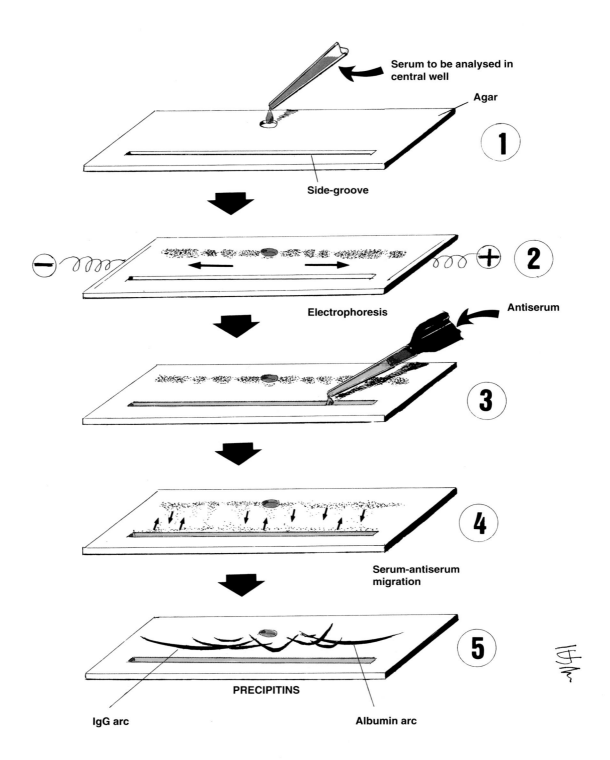

Figure 85

5.4 Immunoelectrophoresis

The principle of immunoelectrophoresis consists of combining electrophoresis with radial immunodiffusion.

The test is carried out as follows (**Figure 85**):

❶ A glass slide, such as a microscope slide, is covered with an agarose layer in which a central well and a longitudinal groove have been punched. A drop of serum to be tested is placed in the well; the groove is reserved for the test antiserum, containing specific antibodies.

❷ An electric field is applied to the agarose layer in order to separate by electrophoresis components of the serum deposited in the well.

❸ At the end of electrophoresis, the patient's serum has been separated into its main fractions, which are then analyzed. Antiserum (usually a mixture of antibodies reacting with the various test serum fractions) is poured into the groove.

❹ Electrophoretically separated serum fractions and test antiserum are allowed to diffuse against each other in the agar layer.

❺ Specific **precipitation arcs** appear at the points where antibodies and serum fractions acting as antigens meet. Each arc corresponds to a well-defined serum fraction. These precipitins are specific. The preparation is stained to allow evaluation of the results.

By means of immunoelectrophoresis, is has been possible to demonstrate the presence of numerous different components in human serum. The various immunoglobulins which are of particular interest in immuno-allergology could also be identified in this way.

COOMBS' TESTS

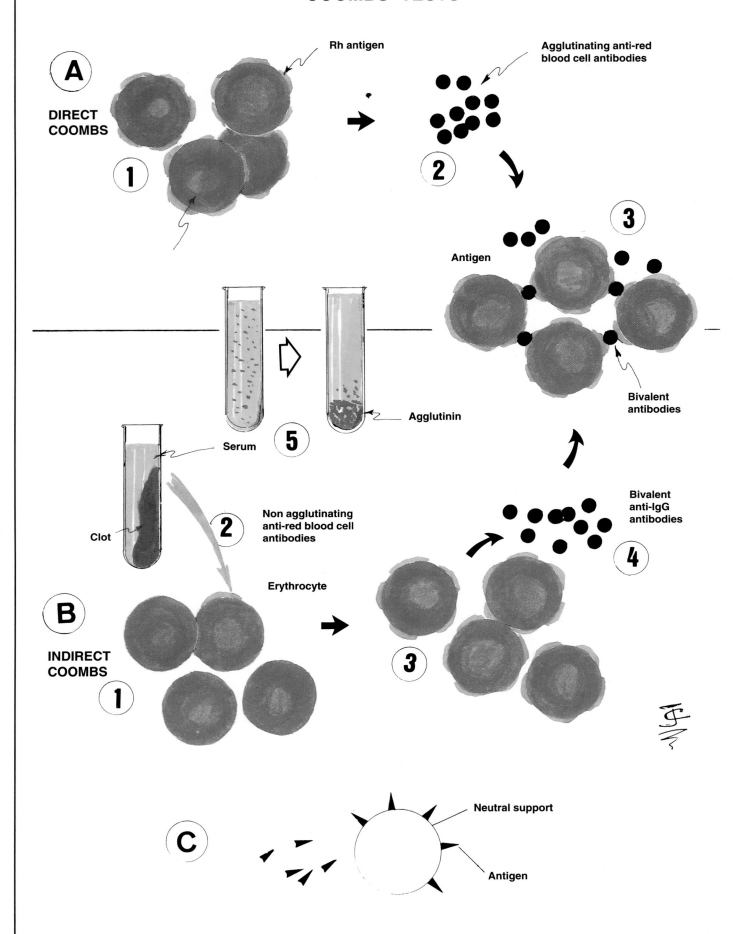

Figure 86

5.5 Agglutination and Passive Hemagglutination

The technique of agglutination is a sensitive method of detecting antibodies, and it has been widely used in immunology. The principle is to fix soluble and invisible antigens on an inert support, such as polystyrene latex or cholesterol microcrystals, etc. Red blood cells may also be used as a support; the technique is then called "hemagglutination." When an antigen is bound to a cell membrane and is part of this membrane, it is said to be a surface antigen. Bivalent antibodies are necessary to obtain agglutination. One frequent diagnostic application of hemagglutination is the **Coombs test**, designed to detect anti-Rh immunization in newborns or infants in whom hemolytic anemia is suspected, or to detect sensitization to the Rh antigen that may have occurred in the mother (the Rh antigen is a membrane antigen present in some red blood cells).

The Direct Coombs' test (Figure 86, A): ❶ Red blood cells with Rh antigen fixed on the surface. ❷ The black circles represent bivalent antibodies (i.e., able to fix two antigenic determinants (epitopes) simultaneously). ❸ The antigen fixed on the red blood cells is brought into contact with the bivalent antibody. Agglutination takes place because the antibodies form real bridges between the red blood cells, producing an Ab-Ag network. In a test tube ❺, this phenomenon is seen as an agglutinate, to the right. Antibodies capable of forming agglutinates are most often immunoglobulins of IgM or IgG class; they were formerly called **agglutinins**.

The Indirect Coombs' test (**Figure 86, B**). Red blood cells ❶ are also used in this test, but initially they do not carry antigen, which is removed from serum after coagulation, e.g. in form of non-agglutinating anti-red blood cell antibodies, functioning as antigen ❷. In ❸, the red blood cells coated with antigen are put in contact ❹ with anti-IgG bivalent antibody. The same phenomenon, i.e., agglutination, is obtained as with the direct Coombs' test.

Figure 86 C shows an **agglutination test** in which red blood cells have been replaced by neutral solid particles such as latex, kaolin, cholesterol microcrystals, etc.

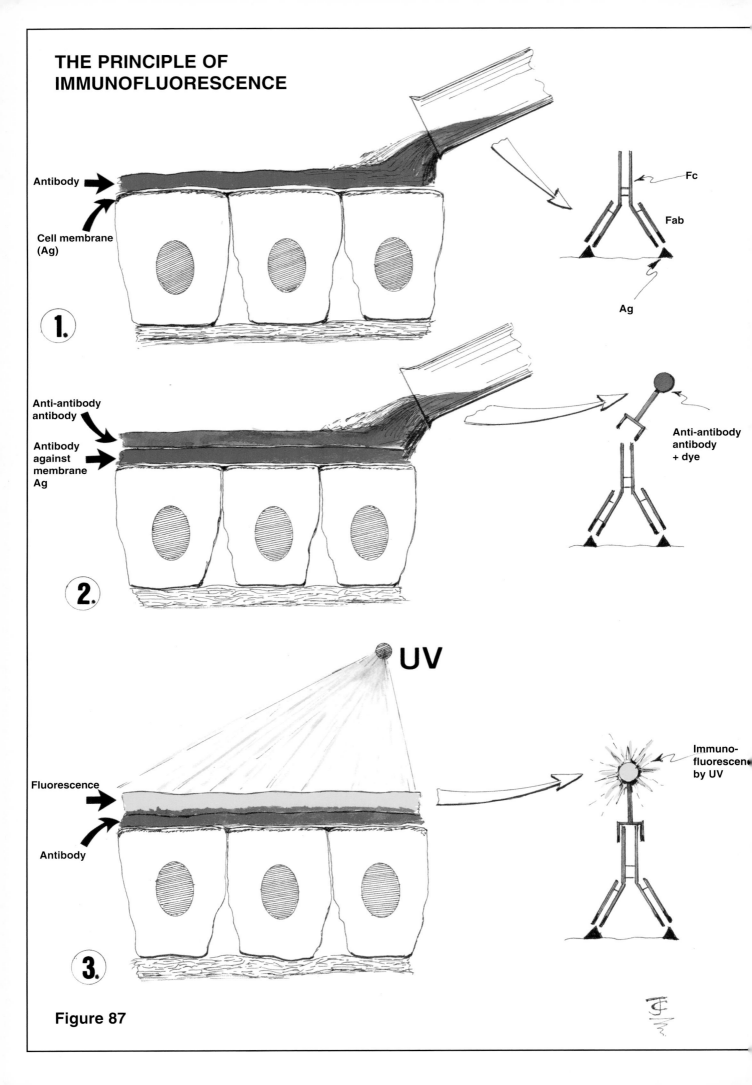

THE PRINCIPLE OF IMMUNOFLUORESCENCE

1.

Antibody

Cell membrane (Ag)

Fc

Fab

Ag

2.

Anti-antibody antibody

Antibody against membrane Ag

Anti-antibody antibody + dye

3.

UV

Fluorescence

Antibody

Immuno-fluorescence by UV

Figure 87

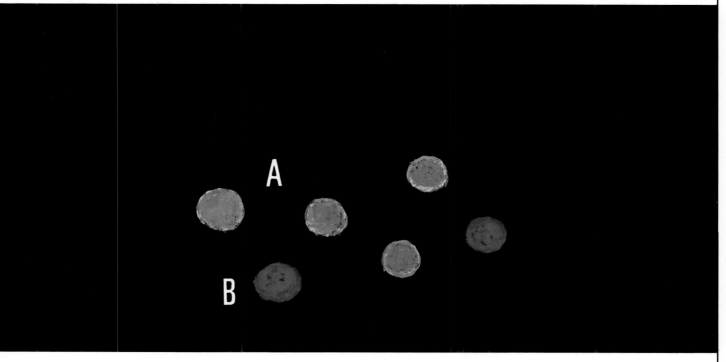

**Lymphocytes which have become fluorescent by means of UV light,
seen on a black microscope background**
A: fluorescein as label
B: rhodamine as label

Figure 88

5.6 Immunofluorescence

Immunofluorescence is a process by which antigen/antibody complexes can be made visible under the microscope. An antibody or antigen may thus be localized and identified in tissue (e. g., in a cryostat section), or on any kind of pathological substance fixed on a microscope slide. γ-Globulins may also be detected on cells in suspension, such as plasmocytes. Microorganisms or antinuclear factors, etc. may be detected in tissues. Selected cells may be sorted out by immunofluorescence, e. g., in leukemia by the flow cytometric (FACS) method.

The preparations are examined under the microscope with ultraviolet light against a black background. The ultraviolet light makes the dyes used fluorescent. These techniques, although delicate, are widely used, especially with monoclonal antibodies. In fact, this amounts to "lighting up" the immunological reaction. The most widely used dyes are fluorescein, yielding a greenish-yellow color, and rhodamine, yielding an orange-red color.

Figure 87 illustrates the principle of immunofluorescence.
In ❶, the antibody is bound specifically by its Fab fragments to the antigens of the cell membrane. In ❷, an anti-antibody Ab binds to the Fc part of the first antibody. In ❸, the preparation is irradiated with ultraviolet light. The anti-antibody Ab to which the special dye is coupled becomes fluorescent.

Figure 88 gives an example of lymphocytes demonstrated by immunofluorescence.

IMMUNOFLUORESCENCE

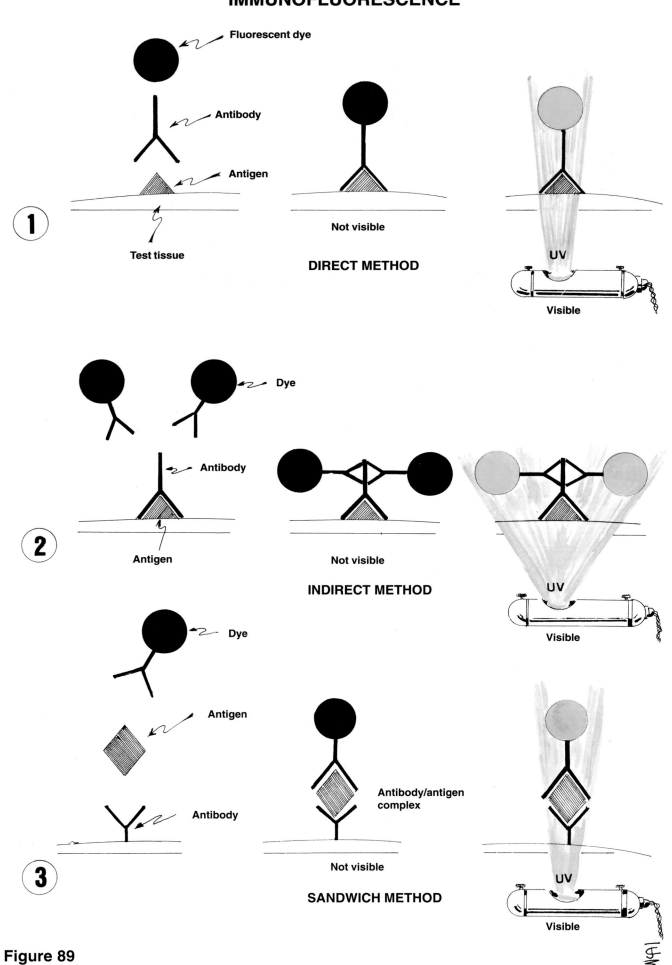

DIRECT METHOD

INDIRECT METHOD

SANDWICH METHOD

Figure 89

We currently use three particular immunofluorescence techniques, illustrated in **Figure 89**:

1. **The Direct Method:** A known antibody directed against a test antigen is labeled with a dye. This antibody is directly applied to the antigen. The reaction is shown in **Figure 89 ❶**. Reading from left to right: elements of the reaction, reaction having taken place but still invisible, reaction made visible by ultraviolet illumination. Special microscopes with appropriate filters are used for immunofluorescence.

2. **The Indirect Technique**: Unmarked antibody is applied directly to the preparation believed to contain the antigen. Next, the antibody-antigen complex is treated with an anti-immunoglobulin serum labeled with dye. Finally, the preparation is placed under the microscope and ultra-violet light is applied. The principles of this reaction are shown in **Figure 89 ❷**. In comparison to the direct variant, the indirect technique yields a more intense fluorescence, since a larger quantity of dye may be fixed to the antigen-antibody complex.

3. **The "Sandwich" Technique (Figure 89 ❸)** is used to locate an intracellular antibody. An unmarked antigen solution is applied to the intracellular antibody to be detected in order to form an antigen-antibody complex. Then, labeled antibody directed against the antigen contained in the antigen/antibody complex is added. Owing to its polyvalent nature (several epitopes), the antigen can simultaneously fix both intracellular and dye-labeled antibodies. Fluorescence appears only, if the labeled antibody has fixed to some intracellular antibody-antigen complex, i. e., if intracellular antibody is present.

ELISA (Sandwich technique)

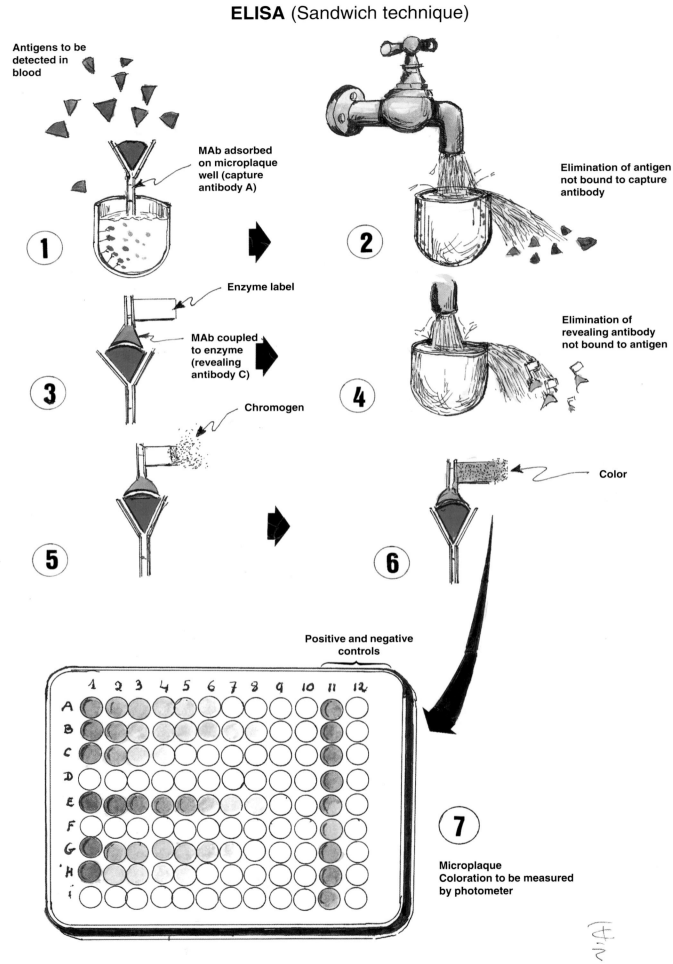

Antigens to be detected in blood

MAb adsorbed on microplaque well (capture antibody A)

1

Elimination of antigen not bound to capture antibody

2

Enzyme label

MAb coupled to enzyme (revealing antibody C)

3

Elimination of revealing antibody not bound to antigen

4

Chromogen

5

Color

6

Positive and negative controls

7

Microplaque Coloration to be measured by photometer

Figure 90

5.7 Chemoluminescence

In principle, antibodies may be labeled with radioactive isotopes (RIA: Radio Immuno Assay, e. g., RAST), with dyes becoming fluorescent under the effect of UV light (Immunofluorescence), by enzymes yielding a colored reaction in the presence of chromogen (ELISA) or by molecules becoming luminescent following a chemical reaction: the latter is the technique of **chemoluminescence.**

In Section 5.11.2, a practical example of an immunological test for the detection of specific IgE, based on chemoluminescence, is shown. Tests relying on chemoluminescence have the advantage of extreme sensitivity but usually require complicated and costly detection equipment.

5.8 Enzyme-Linked Immunosorbent Assay (ELISA)

ELISA is the abbreviation for "Enzyme Linked Immuno Sorbent Assay". Instead of using a radioactive isotope as a label (like in RAST) or a fluorescent dye, as in immunofluorescence, an enzyme (e. g., peroxidase, alkaline phosphatase, etc.) and its substrate (a substance specifically transformed by the enzyme) are used **(Figure 90)**.

The substrate catalyzed by the enzyme reacts with a **chromogen** (substance changing its color according to intensity of the enzyme-substrate reaction).

The most current ELISA technique uses **microplates (Figure 90 ❼)**, in which plastic wells are able to adsorb immunoglobulins on their walls, which constitute a "solid phase" ❶. The technique illustrated in **Figure 90** is called a "sandwich ELISA," since antigen is stuck between two antibody slices. It is used for detecting and quantifying antigens, such as CEA, PSA (tumoral antigens), or antibodies in biological fluids, most often blood.

In a first step, a "capture" antibody **(Ab A)** is adsorbed on the plastic wall of a microplaque, followed by immunological binding of the antigen to be detected ❶. After washing to eliminate molecules not bound to the antibody ❷, a second

antibody called a "revealing antibody" **(Ab C)** is added and binds to the antigen which had been previously captured ❸. Revealing antibody C is coupled (conjugated) to an enzyme (e. g., peroxidase). After washing ❹ to eliminate revealing antibodies not fixed, the substrate and chromogen reacting with the enzyme are added and ❺ bring about a colored reaction, which is often visible to the naked eye ❻ and measurable with a photometer ❼.

An alternative ELISA technique makes use, as a solid phase, of **nitrocellulose strips (Figure 93)**, capable of absorbing antigens or gammaglobulins. The technique illustrated in **Figure 93 B** is a direct method, in which allergen is adsorbed on nitrocellulose and directly detected by an antibody conjugated to an enzyme. Antigens are applied to nitrocellulose as bands or dots **("Immunodot")**.

Nitrocellulose techniques permit direct visual reading without instruments, and are particularly suitable for rapid screening tests, such as pregnancy tests, or the detection of streptococcus infections.

ELISA is used widely in immunology and in medical and pharmaceutical laboratories.

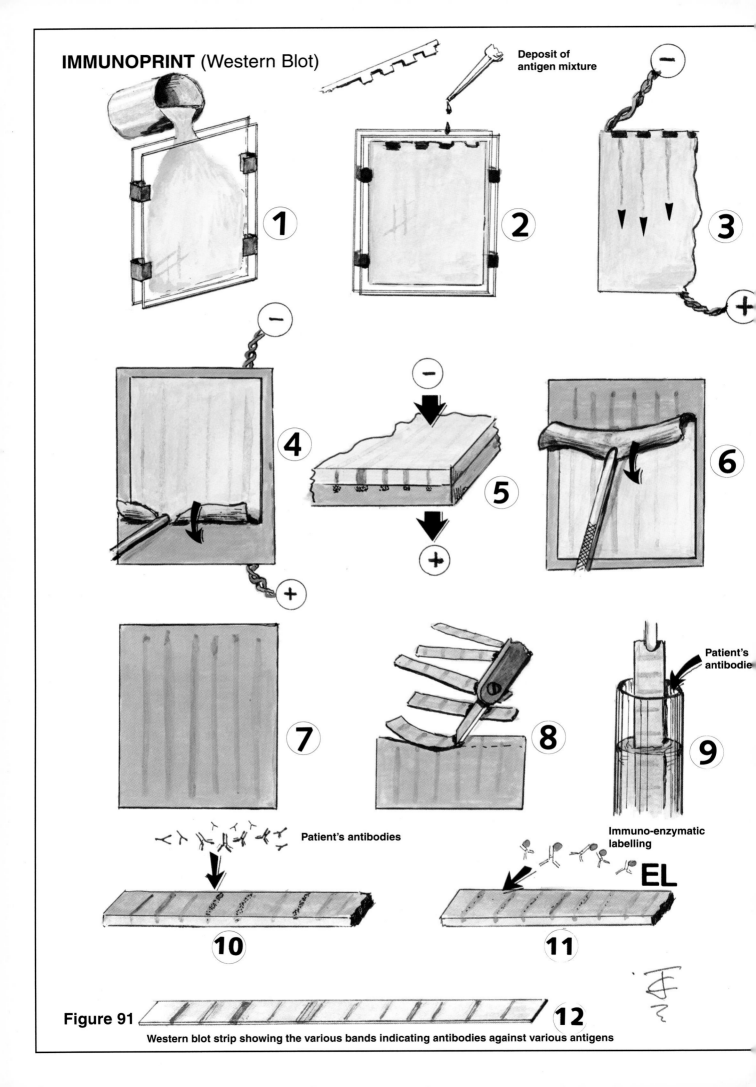

IMMUNOPRINT (Western Blot)

Deposit of antigen mixture

Patient's antibodies

Immuno-enzymatic labelling

EL

Figure 91

Western blot strip showing the various bands indicating antibodies against various antigens

5.9 Immunoprint (Western Blot)

The very sensitive technique, known as **"Western Blot,"** is used increasingly for rapid detection of antibodies of multiple specificities in a liquid phase, or for the analysis of complex mixtures of antigens. It has many applications, the best-known of which is confirmation of the immunological diagnosis of AIDS. An example, which shows how widely this technique may be applied, is the detection of IgE antibodies against latex polypeptides, susceptible to provoke anaphylactic reactions as a result of mere contact with rubber gloves!

The main steps are illustrated in **Figure 91:**
- ❶ Polyacrylamide gel is poured between two glass slides.
- ❷ On one side of the obtained gel layer, grooves are traced with a kind of "comb" and the antigen or antigens corresponding to the antibodies to be detected are deposited therein.
- ❸ The deposited antigens diffuse and separate linearly in the gel by electrophoresis.
- ❹ The gel (yellow) with the diffused and separated antigens is applied on a layer of nitrocellulose (blue).
- ❺ A second electrophoresis is now carried out, from the polyacrylamide to the nitrocellulose layer (from yellow to blue in the figure, as seen in the magnified section). The

antigens migrate only to the surface of the nitrocellulose, hence the name **immunoprint**. When other gel types are used for the incorporation of antigens (e. g., agarose), simple application suffices to transfer electrophoretically separated antigens from gel to nitrocellulose, by capillarity forces.
- ❻ The polyacrylamide gel is removed.
- ❼ Nitrocellulose with antigen bands after electrophoresis. Note that up to this point the bands are invisible.
- ❽ Thin strips of nitrocellulose are cut, so that on each strip the antigens deposited in steps ❷ are present.
- ❾ Nitrocellulose strips containing the separated antigens are incubated with the patient's serum containing antibodies to be identified.
- ❿ Contact between the patient's antibodies and antigens on the nitrocellulose. Immune complexes form wherever an antibody finds its specific antigen.
- ⓫ The ELISA technique, according to the method described above, is used to reveal these immune complexes containing specific antibodies (e. g., anti-HIV antibodies in AIDS). This is carried out with an enzyme-labeled anti-human globulin antibody, followed by addition of substrate and chromogen.
- ⓬ Schematic illustration of a positive immunoprint strip.

167

RAST

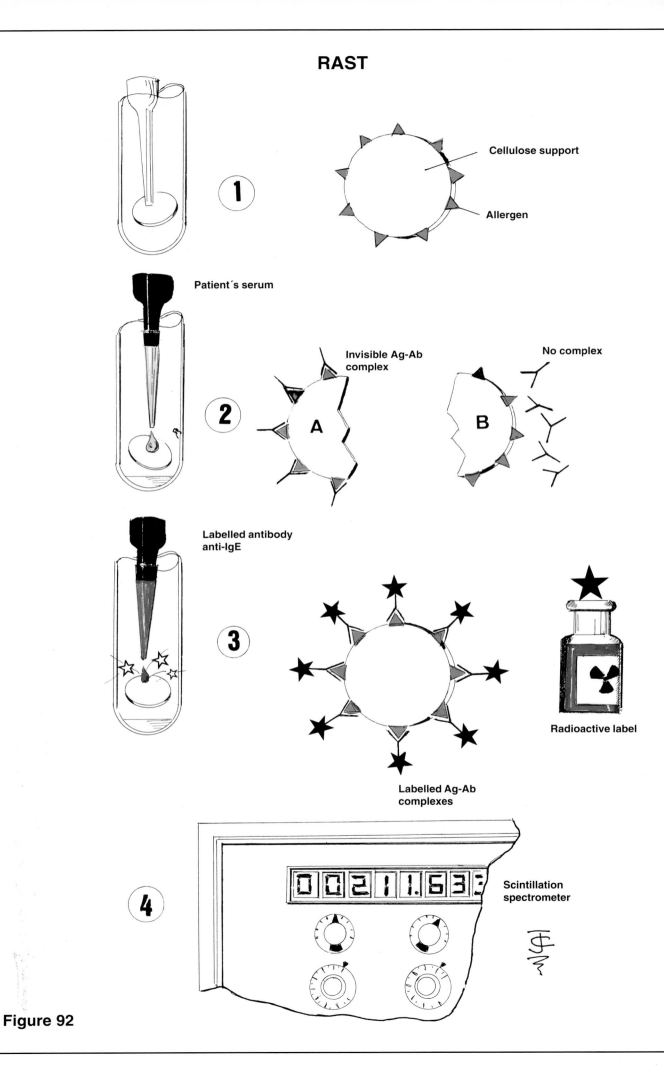

Figure 92

5.10 Determination of Allergen-Specific IgE: RAST/CAP

RAST is the abbreviation for "Radio Allergo Sorbent Test." This ingenious technique has become widely used. It permits detection of IgE antibodies specific to the main allergens in patient sera. Previously, detection of IgE in vitro had been problematic because of its very low serum concentration.

The principle of the technique is as follows **(Figure 92)**: ❶ shows, much magnified, a cellulose disc (actual size: a piece of confetti) to which the manufacturer has "glued" allergens. In general, there is only one variety of allergen per confetti disc, but mixtures may also be used, particularly for preliminary screening tests (e. g., "Phadiatop"®). The confetti is put in a glass tube or a microplate well.

❷ Patient's serum is applied to the disc. If the serum contains IgE antibodies against the corresponding allergen, an antigen-antibody immune complex is formed on the disc surface (❷ A). If there is no specific antibody in the patient's serum, there is no antigen-antibody reaction (❷ B).

The next step permits demonstration of the antigen-antibody complex, which is not visible to the naked eye. For this purpose it is labeled with an anti-IgE antibody directed against the IgE antibody bound in the complex. In ❸, this anti-IgE antibody is represented by a star. It is radioactive, i. e., it emits radiation that may be detected in a liquid scintillation spectrometer. In more recent versions, the anti-IgE antibody may also be labeled with an enzyme and revealed like in the ELISA technique. The results are evaluated according to a "class scale," which is quite sufficient in daily practice.

- Class 0: No radioactivity, i. e., the patient has no specific IgE.
- Class 1 and 2: Fairly weak result, which can be taken into consideration only in a suggestive clinical context.
- Class 3: Moderately positive result.
- Class 4: Strongly positive result.

At present, a new more precise classification in **PRU** (Pharmacia RAST Units, or Protein Related Units) is also used, corresponding to:
- Class 0 =   < 0.35   PRU/ml
- Class 1 =   0.35–0.7   PRU/ml
- Class 2 =   0.7–3.5   PRU/ml
- Class 3 =   3.5–17.5   PRU/ml
- Class 4 =   > 17.5   PRU/ml.

In practice, mostly classes 3 and 4 should be taken into account for clinical diagnosis.

Although RAST is a remarkable technique, it is preferable to start a diagnosis with skin tests or with a serological screening test. RAST may replace skin tests when they are difficult to be carried out, e. g., in infants, or in patients with extensive eczema or intense dermographism. RAST may also be used in cases where allergy tests could be risky, e. g., in anaphylaxis to fish, venoms or latex. Furthermore, in contrast to skin tests, RAST is not affected by antihistamines. It should be noted that RAST does not become positive in practice until the age of about 2–3 years. They may be carried out in infants, especially by capillary blood sampling.

Skin tests and RAST correlate with each other rather well. However, RAST only detects specific IgE in serum, while skin tests assess reactivity of mast cells (see skin tests). RAST may be positive to the one or the other allergen, while the total IgE level is still remaining normal.

In current practice, the principal allergens used in RAST are: Dermatophagoides pteronyssimus and/or farinae house dust mites, grass pollens, cat and dog dander, as well as pollens from Compositae and trees (depending on the region). RAST is also quite useful in allergy to egg white and milk. On the other hand, RAST is not very reliable with moulds and food allergens. RASTs for household dust are of no use at all, and should be abandoned. They test a mixture of large numbers of different allergens, and a positive result does not identify the allergen responsible. In RAST to grass pollens, it is generally sufficient to test one single pollen (e. g., orchard grass) because of wide cross allergenicity between various grass pollen allergens.

An improved variant of the RAST technique has recently been commercialized. It consists of replacing the disc carrying the antigen with a micro-sponge capable of fixing a much larger amount of allergen. This variation is called the **CAP test**. The principle is the same as in RAST, using enzyme-labeled anti-IgE antibodies. The test is, however, more sensitive and results are expressed in 6 PRU classes. Various other techniques for the detection of specific IgE, based on similar immunological or slightly modified principles have appeared during recent years, such as the detection of allergens in liquid phase (ALASTAT), and by chemoluminescence (MAGIC-LITE).

DETERMINATION OF ALLERGEN SPECIFIC IgE

A. PAPER STRIPS (Quidel Test)

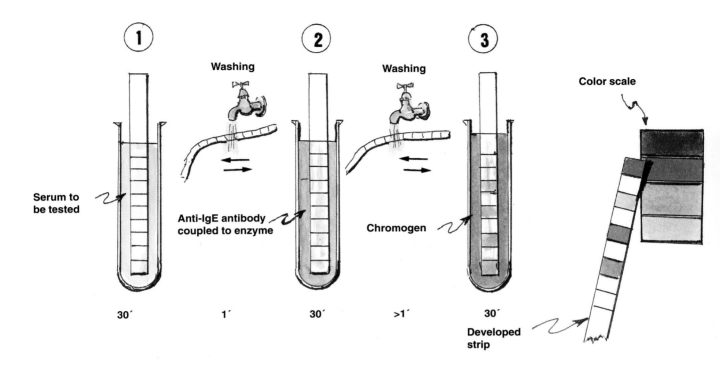

B. NITROCELLULOSE STRIPS (Immunodot CMG Test)

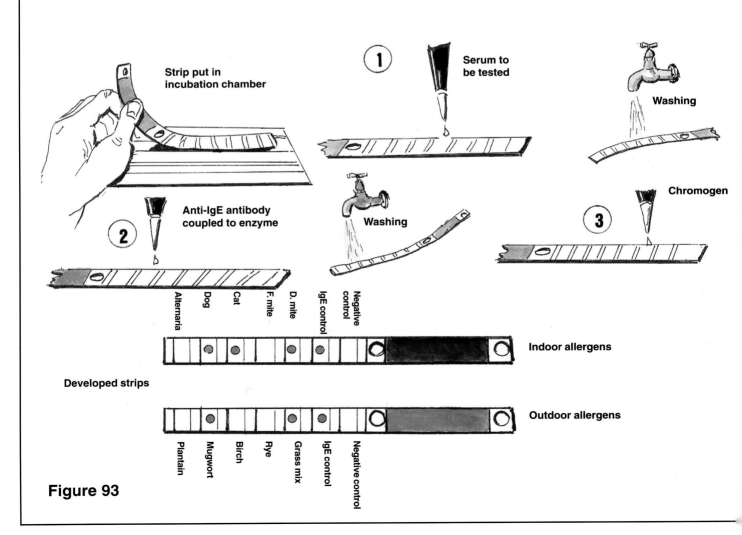

Figure 93

5.11 Other Techniques for IgE Determination

5.11.1 Strip techniques

To facilitate detection of allergies by practitioners who are usually not familiar with the tedious skin test procedures, simpler technologies have been developed in recent years. These tests may be performed in medical practices or simple laboratories and do not require costly instrument investments, such as are involved with the RAST or CAP techniques.

These tests use paper **(Figure 93 A)** or nitrocellulose **(Figure 93 B)** strips on which allergen extracts are applied in form of bands or dots. After incubation of the strip with patient's serum containing IgE specific for the one or the other allergen, IgE antibodies having fixed to the strip are revealed by an enzyme-labeled anti-IgE antibody, like in ELISA. Color reactions produced by reaction of the enzyme with the appropriate substrate and chromogen permits us to read the reaction with the naked eye, and to estimate its intensity, in various class divisions, like in more complicated techniques.

Thus, it is possible in one single manipulation to detect the main allergens to which a patient might be sensitized.

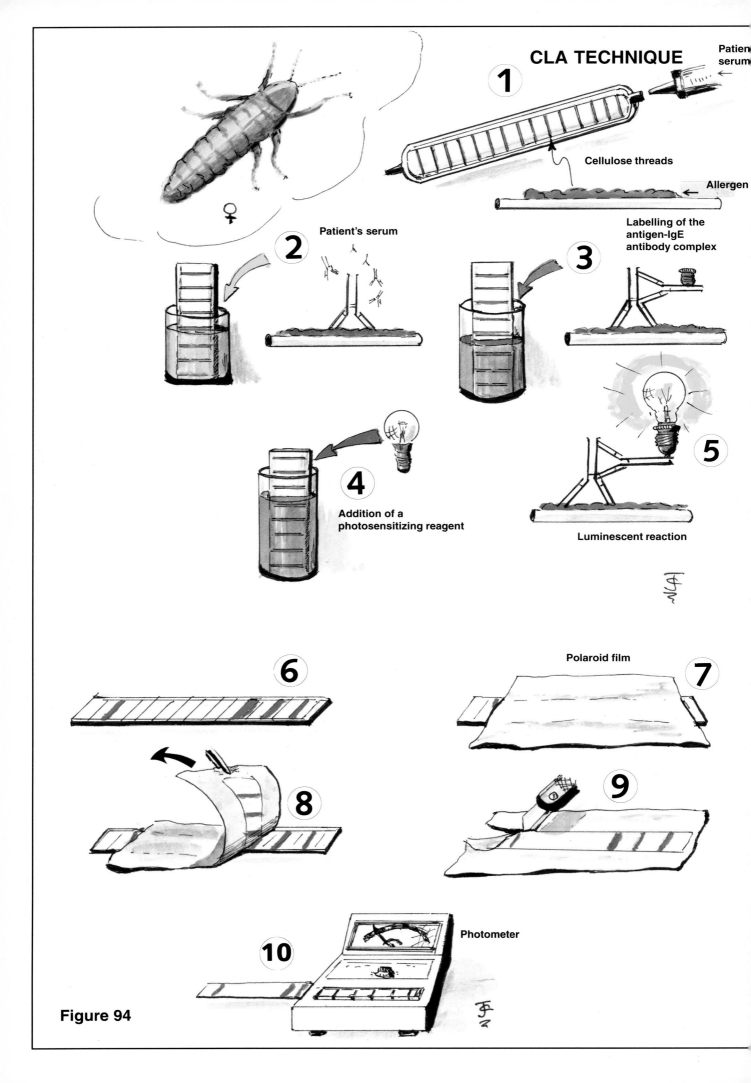

CLA TECHNIQUE

1 — Patient's serum / Cellulose threads / Allergen

Labelling of the antigen-IgE antibody complex

2 — Patient's serum

3

4 — Addition of a photosensitizing reagent

5 — Luminescent reaction

6

7 — Polaroid film

8

9

10 — Photometer

Figure 94

5.11.2 CLA technique (chemoluminescent assay)

The principle of this sophisticated method is similar to that of RAST and ELISA, except that the antigen-IgE reaction is made visible by an enzyme reaction visualized by **chemoluminescence**, rather than by radioactive labeling or by a colorimetric reaction. This approach is also used for the diagnosis of allergies mediated by IgE.

Bioluminescence is a known phenomenon in certain bacteria and mollusks and, in particular, in the glow-worm (Lampyris noctiluca). Luciferin in these insect bodies becomes luminescent, owing to an enzyme called luciferase. Bioluminescence is used in various biochemical analyses, in particular for determining dosages of ATP.

Figure 94 illustrates the CLA technique, showing at the top, on the left, a female glow-worm (females produce the strongest luminescence, apparently to attract males).

– ❶ 36 cellulose threads are stretched out perpendicularly in an incubation pipette. Each thread has been impregnated with an allergen. The allergen(e. g., grass pollen), is shown on its thread in green.

– ❷ Patient serum suspected of containing anti-pollen IgE is introduced into the pipette. Specific IgE combines with antigen fixed to the cellulose threads.

– ❸ Anti-IgE IgG labeled with an enzyme (represented by a light bulb) is added. Up to this point, the phenomenon is invisible to the naked eye.

– ❹ Addition of a photosensitizing reagent lights up the system.

– ❺ The Ag-IgE/anti-IgE antibody complex (symbolized by the lit electric bulb).

– ❻ Since this luminescence is too weak to be visible to the naked eye, Polaroid photographic paper ❼ is applied. In ❽, the paper is stripped off after suitable time of exposure.

– ❾ The photographed strip is cut out and read using a photometer, which indicates positivity and density of the luminescence achieved.

ROSETTES

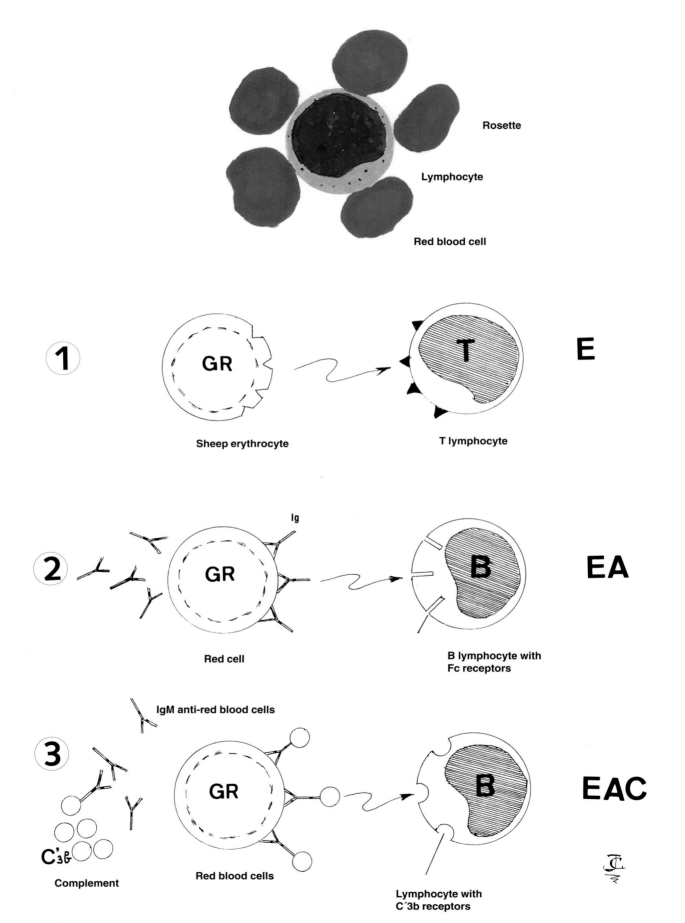

Rosette

Lymphocyte

Red blood cell

1 Sheep erythrocyte → T lymphocyte **E**

GR → T

2 Red cell → B lymphocyte with Fc receptors **EA**

Ig

GR → B

3 IgM anti-red blood cells

C'₃b Complement

Red blood cells

GR → B

Lymphocyte with C'3b receptors **EAC**

Figure 95

5.12 Rosette Tests

Rosette tests were the first techniques which permitted us to distinguish and separate various lymphocyte subpopulations.

The classical microscope picture of a "rosette" is formed by a lymphocyte or another cell to the membrane of which several red blood cells, at least four or five, have attached, forming the image of "rose petals."

There are several types of rosettes, as seen in **Figure 95**, the main ones being:

- ❶ Human T lymphocytes have specific receptors for sheep red blood cells (erythrocytes) on their surface. If T lymphocytes and sheep erythrocytes are brought into contact, they form a rosette known as **E rosette** (E for erythrocyte).

- ❷ B lymphocytes and macrophages, in addition to K cells and certain T lymphocytes, have surface receptors for Fc fragments of IgG. If these cells are placed in contact with erythrocytes incubated with anti-erythrocyte IgG, **EA rosettes** (**E** for erythrocyte and **A** for antibody) or **Fc rosettes** are obtained.

- ❸ B lymphocytes, monocytes, and polynuclears also have receptors for certain complement factors, particularly for C'3b. Erythrocytes incubated with anti-erythrocyte IgM and complement may form rosettes in the presence of such cells. These are called **EAC rosettes** (**E** for erythrocyte, **A** for antibody, and **C** for complement).

Erythrocytes can also act as support: if lymphocytes possess membrane structures specific to an antigen, they fix erythrocytes coated with this antigen. The antigen is "glued" artificially to the erythrocytes beforehand.

Rheumatoid rosette. Rheumatoid factor is an IgM auto-antibody directed against the patient's IgG (Fc fragment). Lymphocytes which are carrying this IgM on their surface and put in contact with erythrocytes incubated with antihuman IgG will form rosettes. It turns out that 70% of patients suffering from rheumatoid arthritis are carriers of rheumatoid factors.

It remains to be said that rosettes techniques are delicate and provide many opportunities for making mistakes. As a result, in practice they have been, for analytical purposes, practically replaced by flux cytometry (see 5.14). Rosette techniques may, however, still be useful in order to sort lymphocyte subpopulations by immunoadsorption with antibodies adhering to some solid phase, or to magnetic beads. This involves so-called "panning" techniques.

LYMPHOBLAST TRANSFORMATION TEST

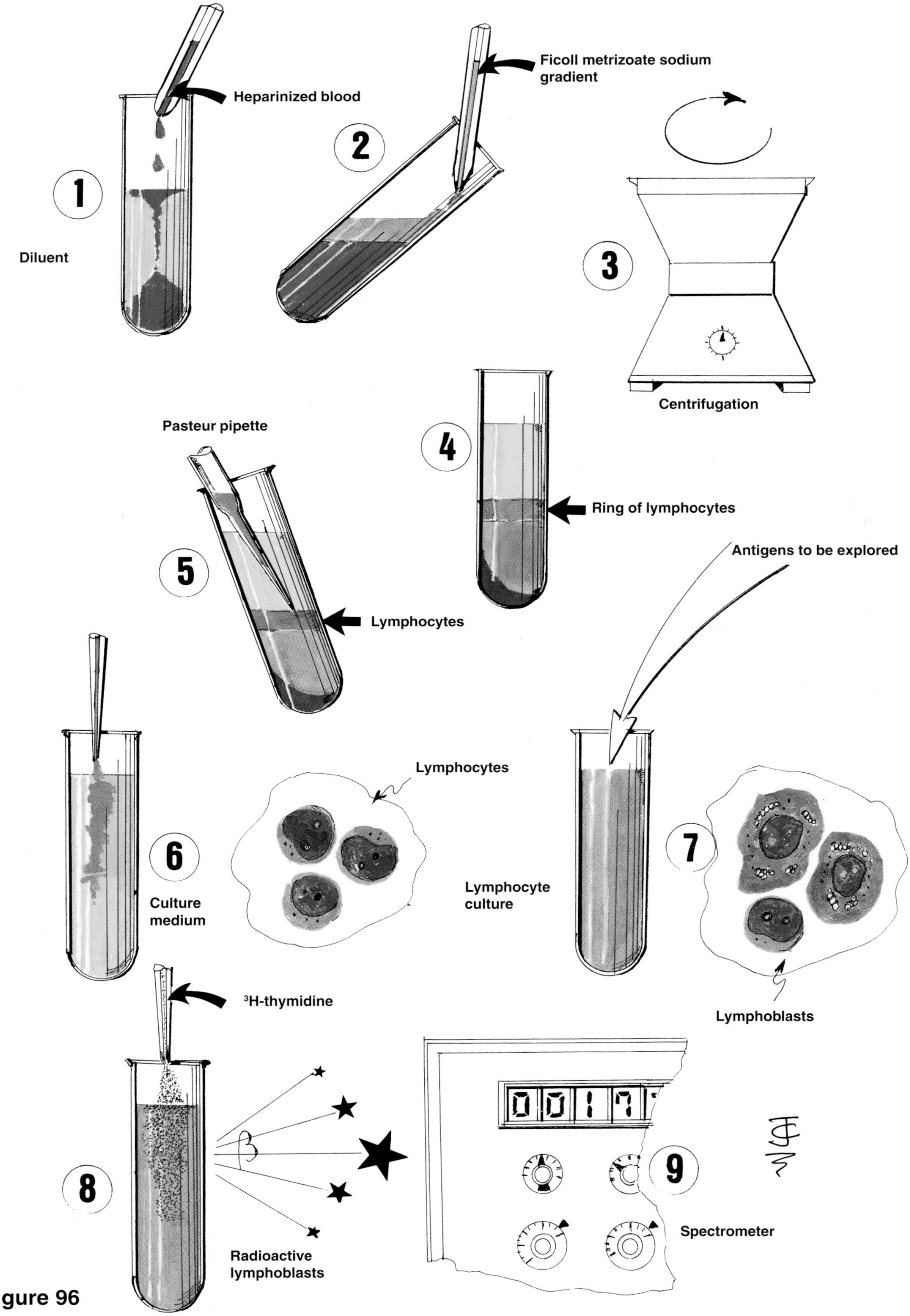

Figure 96

5.13 Lymphocyte Proliferation Test

This technique consists of placing lymphocytes in vitro in contact with an antigen to which they might be sensitive. If the reaction is positive, the lymphocyte is transformed into a **lymphoblast**, which is easily recognized under the microscope.

The method is represented schematically in **Figure 96:**
- In ❶, heparinized blood is placed in diluent, e. g., saline.
- In ❷, a special density gradient medium for centrifuging erythrocytes and polymorphonuclear cells (Ficoll/metrizoate sodium) is added to the diluted blood and the mixture is centrifuged ❸.
- In ❹, the various fractions obtained by centrifugation are seen: in yellow the diluent, in orange the lymphocytes, in green the Ficoll Metrizoate medium, and in dark red the erythrocytes and polymorphonuclears.
- In ❺, lymphocytes are sucked up with a Pasteur pipette and placed in a special culture medium ❻. In ❼ the antigen to be tested, or a so-called mitogenic substance, which provokes the same cellular proliferation, but in a non-specific manner (phytohemagglutinin – PHA), is added. The culture is left then to incubate for 3–7 days at 37°C. Under the effect of specific antigen or of PHA, the lymphocytes transform into lymphoblasts ❼, which is the stage preceding cell division and proliferation, hence the name "lymphocyte proliferation technique"

The lymphoblasts may be counted under the microscope, a difficult and tedious procedure which has been practically abandoned. Nowadays, radioactive thymidine is added ❽, which is taken up exclusively by the lymphoblasts. The DNA of lymphoblasts thus becomes radioactive, and this radioactivity may be measured ❾ in a liquid scintillation spectrometer. The radioactivity increases in proportion to the number of lymphoblasts, hence only a simple calculation remains to be done.

The lymphocyte proliferation technique is used mainly in research or for evaluating immune competence, and only seldom in allergological practice (sometimes in attempts to detect a drug allergy).

Lymphocyte stimulation caused by antigens or mitogens may manifest itself earlier than lymphoblast proliferation in culture, which needs at least 3 days. Already after 24 to 48 hours it is possible to determine the appearance of some receptors on the membrane of stimulated lymphocytes, for example receptors for interleukin 2: IL-2R. These receptors may be detected by immunofluorescence under the microscope or by FACS. In the culture medium of stimulated lymphocytes, lymphokines appear, such as IL-2, γ-interferon, which may be detected by ELISA techniques.

FLOW CYTOMETRY (FACS)

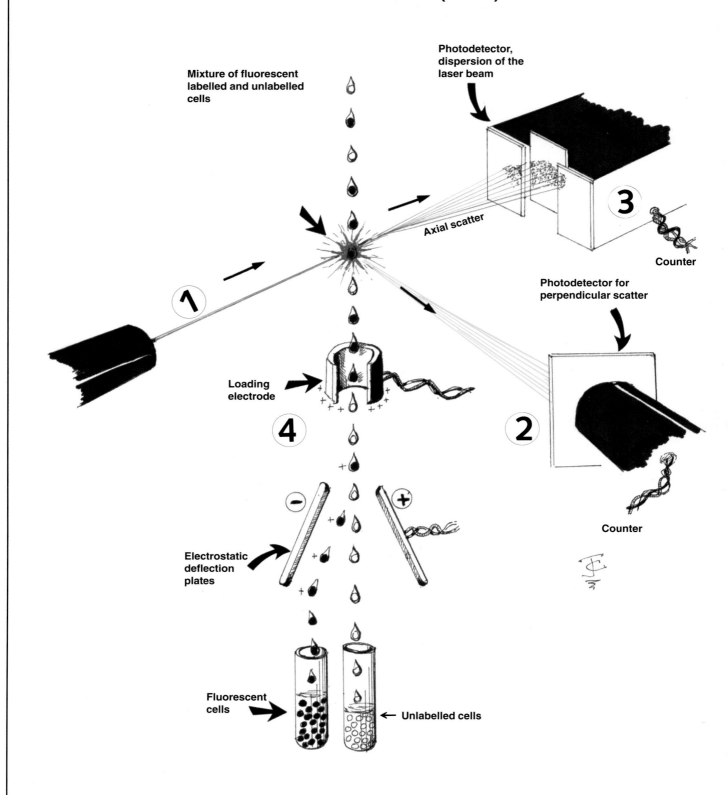

Mixture of fluorescent labelled and unlabelled cells

Photodetector, dispersion of the laser beam

Axial scatter

① ③

Counter

Photodetector for perpendicular scatter

②

Counter

Loading electrode

④

Electrostatic deflection plates

− +

Fluorescent cells

Unlabelled cells

Figure 97

CELL ANALYSIS BY FACS

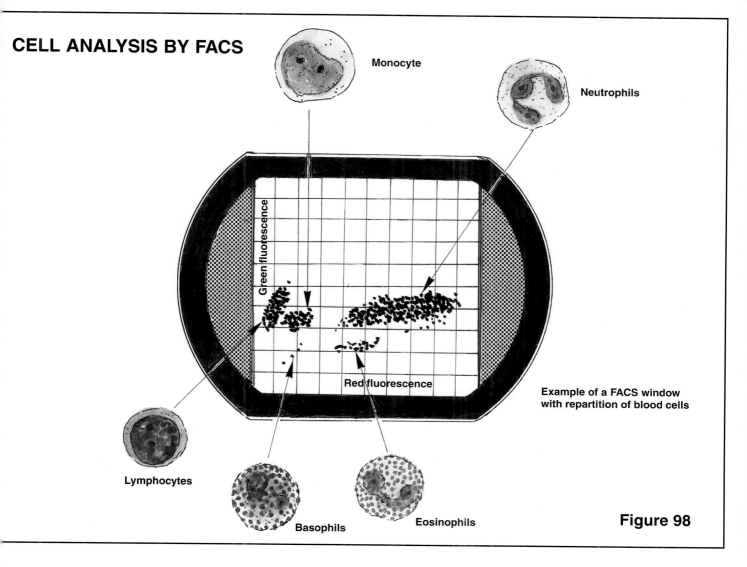

Monocyte

Neutrophils

Green fluorescence

Red fluorescence

Example of a FACS window
with repartition of blood cells

Lymphocytes

Basophils

Eosinophils

Figure 98

5.14 Flow Cytometry (FACS)

This analytical technique is based on immunofluorescence. The treated cells are analyzed or sorted according to their degree of fluorescence by an instrument called a FACS (Fluorescence Activated Cell Sorter).

The principle of the FACS is relatively straightforward: a suspension of cells treated with MAbs marked with a fluorochrome (or even with several fluorochromes possessing different spectra) is carried by a jet of saline diluent through a very fine capillary. This flow of cells is subjected to high-frequency vibrations produced by a piezoelectric crystal vibrator. The jet is thus fractionated into thousands of droplets (400,000/sec), each containing in principle a single cell.

The column of droplets crosses a laser beam oriented perpendicularly to it **(Figure 97 ❶)**. The cell labeled with fluorochrome contained in the droplet then becomes fluorescent, which does not occur with cells that have not fixed a specific MAb. The fluorescence (perpendicular scatter) ❷ is detected by an optical system. The received signals are transformed into electrical impulses, which are then analyzed by computer. Another detector ❸, situated on the same axis as the laser beam (axial scatter), measures cell dispersion. This is proportional to the cell volume. In this way, a two-dimensional analysis of cell populations may be performed **(Figure 98)**.

The FACS enables us to distinguish living from dead cells, since their light dispersion is quite different. Rare cells (e. g., tumor cells, cells with abnormal chromosomes, etc.) may also be detected in a blood cell population, an impossible task with a microscope. With this technique it also becomes possible to isolate B lymphocytes, to measure the CD4/CD8 ratio in AIDS, to identify HLA carrying cells in grafts, etc. Results are nicely visible on a TV monitor and the graphs obtained **(Figure 98)** may be electronically registered and printed.

For cellular selection and isolation **("sorting"),** electrically charged droplets ❹ are instantly and selectively attracted by an electrode, according to data obtained from the laser (fluorescence and volume). The cells next pass between two electrostatic plates and are deviated according to their charge ❺. The system is regulated in such a manner that cells fall into different tubes depending on their characteristics. In this way, a considerable number of cells (5,000–10,000/sec) may be sorted individually and very rapidly. Certain devices allow individual seeding of wells in microplates, e. g., for cell cloning, isolating an hybridoma, etc.

179

MEDIATOR RELEASE TESTS

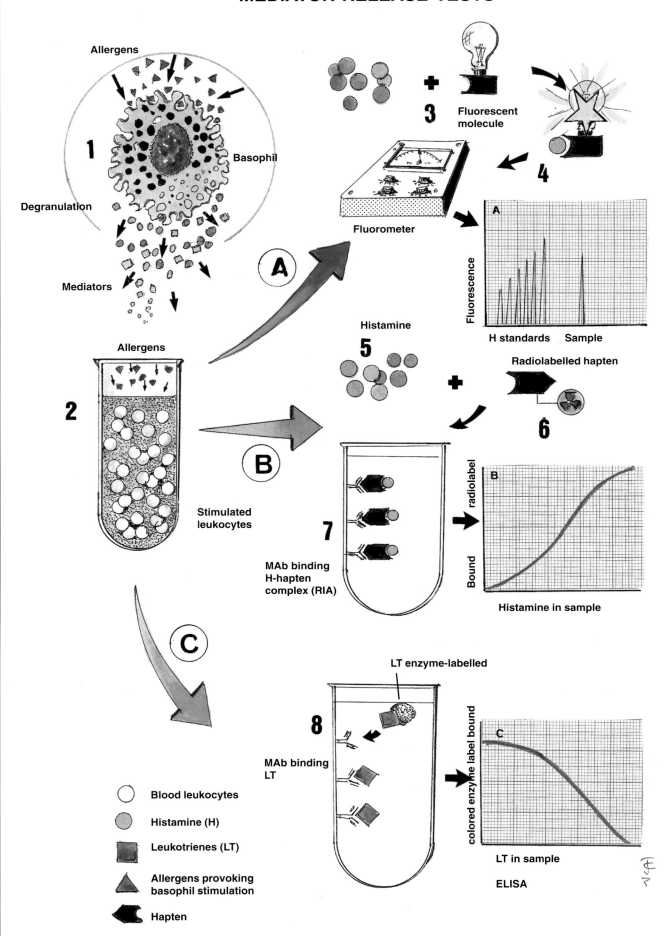

Figure 99

5.15 Release Tests for Cellular Mediators

Tests based on the determination of free IgE in serum yield only indirect information concerning the existence of allergies: not free IgE antibodies, but those bound to the membranes of mast cells and basophils, are responsible for cell activation and the release of mediators, such as histamine or leukotrienes. Finally, these mediators are the ones responsible for clinical allergic symptoms. In addition, specific IgE antibody levels measured in serum do not correlate exactly, on an individual basis, with the severity of clinical symptoms. Some patients may possess much IgE but exhibit relatively few symptoms, while others may have relatively little IgE but severe symptoms. This is due to the fact that cellular reactivity and capacity to release mediators varies considerably from one individual to the other, but also in the same individual, depending on the time period.

Therefore, in addition to allergen specific antibodies, another variable is the capacity to produce mediators (**"releasibility"**). It has become apparent that certain cytokines, in particular IL-3, IL-5 and GM-CSF (see 1.12.6) have a major influence on this parameter.

As a result, various tests which allow us to evaluate mediator release upon allergen contact have been developed. A first test, widely used in research, is **histamine release (Figure 99)**. In this approach blood leukocytes containing basophils loaded with histamine are brought in contact with an incriminated allergen. When specific IgE is present for that allergen on the membrane of basophils, the reaction will be followed by degranulation and histamine re-

lease. This reaction may be intensified by addition of a small amount of cytokine, for example, IL-3. We can detect released histamine in cell supernatants by automated fluorimetry **(Figure 99, A)**, because histamine reacts relatively specific with certain fluorescent chemicals. Another possibility is immunochemical analysis, after chemical conjugation of histamine with another chemical molecule (hapten) against which a monoclonal antibody has been produced **(Figure 99, B)**. This "detour" was needed, since it has proven difficult to produce antibodies exactly specific for histamine, which is a very small molecule.

Another possibility is to assess **leukotriene production,** particularly LTC4 and its metabolites LTD4 and LTE4 during allergic in vitro reactions. Leukotrienes may be analyzed thanks to a specific monoclonal antibody in immunochemical reactions of the ELISA type. In this assay, detection is achieved through competitive displacement by native leukotrienes, produced in cell supernatants, of a fixed amount of enzyme labeled LTD4 bound to tube wall adsorbed antileukotriene MAb **(Figure 99, C).**

Aside from physiopathological allergy research, these cellular mediator release tests have increasing clinical indications, such as allergy diagnosis in infants, monitoring of specific immunotherapy, and the indication of immunotherapy in cases where there are discrepancies between the patient's history, serology and skin tests. Finally, these tests may yield useful results in allergies and pseudo-allergies to drugs.

QUICK TEST FOR TUBERCULOSIS DETECTION

THE CLASSICAL TECHNIQUES

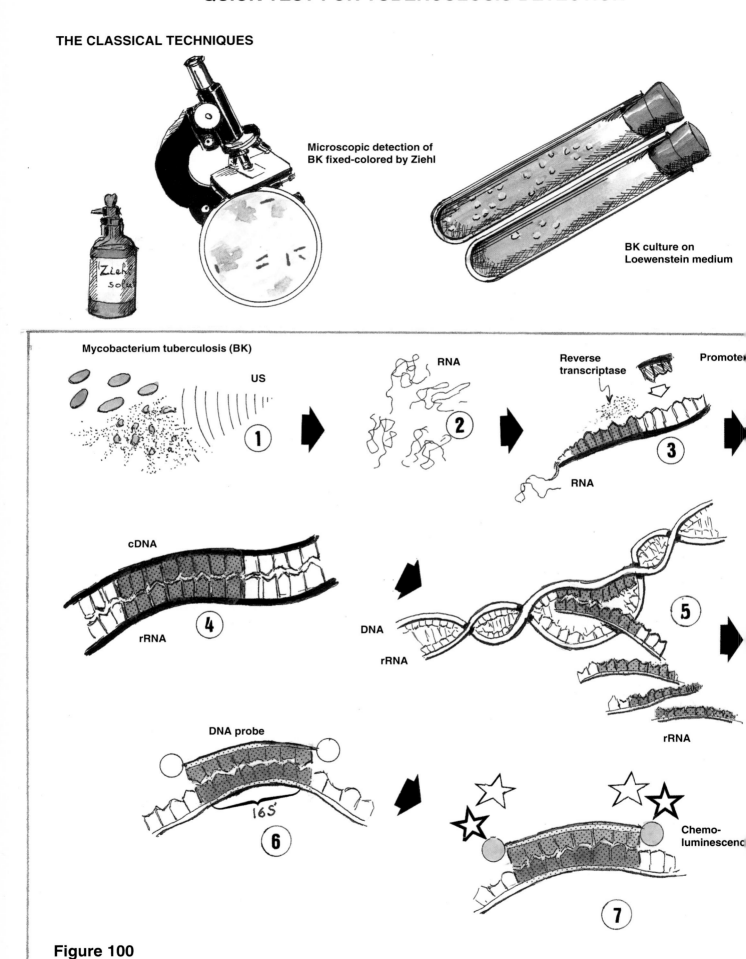

Microscopic detection of
BK fixed-colored by Ziehl

BK culture on
Loewenstein medium

Mycobacterium tuberculosis (BK)

US

①

RNA

②

Reverse
transcriptase

Promoter

RNA

③

cDNA

rRNA

④

DNA

rRNA

⑤

rRNA

DNA probe

16S'

⑥

Chemo-
luminescence

⑦

Figure 100

5.16 Molecular Biology, a Twin Sister of Immunology. A Quick Test for Detection of Tuberculosis

Genetic engineering, molecular biology and immunology are increasingly associated; they have really become twin sisters. For this reason, it is often no longer possible to discuss one technology without mentioning the other, in order to compare, combine or exchange them. A particularly striking example is a new quick test for **detection of tuberculosis** (GEN-PROBE).

Tuberculosis, which was thought to be almost eradicated, has recently become more prevalent, fostered by AIDS, poverty, and by various conflicts, particularly in Africa.

Classical diagnostic techniques, such as microscopic detection of mycobacteria and culture remain valid, but are not always practical, and in any case are much too slow, since 4 to 6 weeks are needed for cultures on Loewenstein medium or derived media. Early diagnosis is particularly important in cases of "closed" tuberculosis, which yield few mycobacteria. These forms are the most frequent in Africa: meningitis, pleurisy, bone or lymph node tuberculosis, renal tuberculosis, etc. The earlier that treatment can begin, the easier it is to cure tuberculosis.

The new GEN-PROBE test enables us to make a diagnosis of tuberculosis in less than four hours, based theoretically on one bacterium. It is based, on the one hand, on hybridization with a small segment of the BK (Koch Bacillus) and, on the other hand, on considerable amplification in the number of targeted gene products (RNAr). **Figure 100** summarizes the principles of this technique:

In ❶, the BK potentially present in a biological sample are lysed by ultrasound **(US)** in order to disrupt their thick walls and to permit the release of RNA. **The target of the test is ribosomal RNA (RNAr) of the BK,** in fact its 16S moiety. RNA is a better target, as it is present in much larger amounts than DNA ❷. These RNAr serve as a template for producing ❸ other copies translated in DNA **(DNAc)**. They also help align and join nucleotides, thanks to certain specific enzymes, including the reverse transcriptase **(TR)** which effects a very important multiplication process, aligning and joining nucleotides.

This mechanism is induced by a "promoter," formed from a few nucleotides. Symbolized in red is the portion of the gene product to analyze, a subunit of RNAr (16 S).

In ❹–❺ RNAr-DNAc hybridization makes it possible to produce numerous copies (millions!) in a few cycles at fixed temperature, and thereby to increase considerably the sensitivity of the test.

Detection of the copies will occur by hybridization of the 16 S RNAr subunits with a DNA probe (green) labeled with acridinium ester ❻ **(EA)**. Measurement is effected by direct chemoluminescence **(CL)**, in that a reagent liberating energy, manifested by light emission, is added. The latter will be detected and registered by a photomultiplier.

Rapid diagnosis of tuberculosis may result in important benefits, and thereby justify the still relatively high cost of such diagnostic techniques.

Index

IgG 49
IgM 49
immunoglobulin classes 49
immunological tolerance 93
immunoscintigraphy 59
immunosuppressive therapy 131
interferon 41
interleukins 41
intrinsic asthma 101

K

K or killer lymphocytes 15
Kaposi's sarcoma 117

L

Langerhans cells 13, 35
late phase reaction 89, 105
leukotrienes 79, 103, 181
lymph nodes 19
lympho-monocytic inflammation 91
lymphoblast 177
lymphocyte proliferation test 177
lymphokines 13, 41

M

macrophages 35
major basic protein (MBP) 11
major histocompatibility complex (MHC) 124
malaria 141
mast cells 77
migration inhibition factor (MIF) 87
monoclonal antibodies 57
monocytes 13
mucosal mast cells (MMC) 13

N

neutrophils 3, 7
nitrocellulose strips 165
normodense eosinophils 11

O

opsonization 37
orchitis 133

P

PAF 103
patch test 111
PCR (Polymerase Chain reaction) 69
Peyer's patches 23
phytohemagglutinin PHA 177
plasmocytes 15, 45
platelet-activating factor 79

pollinosis 100
polyps 101
precipitins 151
prick test 111
primary response 51
priming phenomenon 43, 89
prostaglandins 79, 103
pseudo-allergic reactions 43, 89
pyogenic inflammation 91

R

RAST 169
recognition of self 17
recombinant allergens 137
releasibility 181
repertoire cloning 67
rosette tests 175

S

scratch test 111
secondary response 51
secretory IgA 49
serotherapy 139
sorting, cell 179
spleen 21
strip techniques 171
sympathetic ophthalmia 133

T

T cell receptor (TCR) 39
T lymphocytes 13, 31
Th lymphocytes 13
Th1 lymphocytes 112
Th2 lymphocytes 112
theophylline 113
thoracic duct 25
thymus 17
tissue mast cells (CTMC) 13
TNF (Tumor Necrosis Factor) 41
Ts lymphocytes 13
tuberculosis 183
tumoral antigens 143

U

urticaria 108

V

vaccination 139

W

Western Blot 167
Wiskott-Aldrich syndrome 114